DIAGNOSTIC AUDIOLOGY POCKET GUIDE

Evaluation of Hearing, Tinnitus, and Middle Ear Function

Editor-in-Chief for Audiology
Brad A. Stach, PhD

DIAGNOSTIC AUDIOLOGY POCKET GUIDE

Evaluation of Hearing, Tinnitus, and Middle Ear Function

James Steiger, PhD
Erin L. Miller, AuD

PLURAL PUBLISHING INC.

PLURAL PUBLISHING
INC.

5521 Ruffin Road
San Diego, CA 92123

e-mail: info@pluralpublishing.com
Website: http://www.pluralpublishing.com

FSC
www.fsc.org
MIX
Paper from responsible sources
FSC® C011935

Typeset in 11/13 Garamond Book by Flanagan's Publishing Service, Inc.
Printed in the United States of America by McNaughton & Gunn, Inc.

Library of Congress Cataloging-in-Publication Data

Names: Steiger, James, author. | Miller, Erin L., author.
Title: Diagnostic audiology pocket guide : evaluation of hearing, tinnitus, and middle ear function / James Steiger, Erin L. Miller.
Description: San Diego, CA : Plural, [2017] | Includes bibliographical references and index.
Identifiers: LCCN 2016056743| ISBN 9781944883973 (alk. paper) | ISBN 1944883975 (alk. paper)
Subjects: | MESH: Audiometry—methods | Hearing Disorders—diagnosis | Handbooks
Classification: LCC RF294 | NLM WV 39 | DDC 617.8/075—dc23
LC record available at https://lccn.loc.gov/2016056743

Contents

Preface

This text is intended for use as a lab-coat pocket reference, aimed first at AuD students and recent graduates, though more experienced audiologists might also benefit from having easy access to the information herein. Chapters 1 through 17 of this text pertain to specific tests or test groupings. Those chapters are followed by Chapters 18 through 25 on disorders. Chapter 26 is comprised of example audiograms. Finally, Chapter 27 provides information on medical referral decision making. We hope that the audiologist that has this text in his or her lab-coat pocket will have a valuable and quick reference for every day audiologic diagnosis and referral.

Acknowledgments

The authors thank the many Northeast Ohio AuD Consortium students who have contributed to this text by teaching us through their presentations in grand rounds and clinical learning labs. Special thanks to Kate Weatherholt for her technical help and Kaylee Miller for her drafting, editing, and research. Finally, Emily Rospert deserves special thanks; she did all of the above and more.

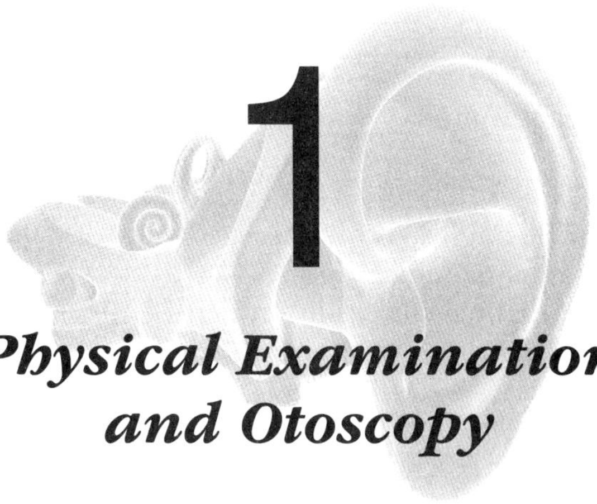

1 Physical Examination and Otoscopy

OVERVIEW

Our purpose in this short overview is twofold. First, we provide tips for conducting otoscopy safely and effectively, and for purchasing the equipment to facilitate those efforts. Second, we describe normal findings and give a few examples of abnormalities that are commonly seen.

OTOSCOPES

The most commonly used otoscopes are portable. Included in the head of the otoscope is a magnifying lens, a light source with an on/off button, and an attachment for speculum. Specula come in various sizes for different ear canal apertures. Portable units are powered by batteries located in the handle. Typically, these batteries can be recharged by plugging the handle into an electrical outlet.

Otoscope Types

- Standard (Figure 1–1)
- Wide-angle: allows enlarged view of entire tympanic membrane (Figure 1–2)
- Operating: allows insertion of tools into ear canal to extract cerumen or foreign bodies
- Video: allows patient and family to observe, captures images (Figure 1–3)

Illumination

There are several types of illumination to choose from, each having unique characteristics.

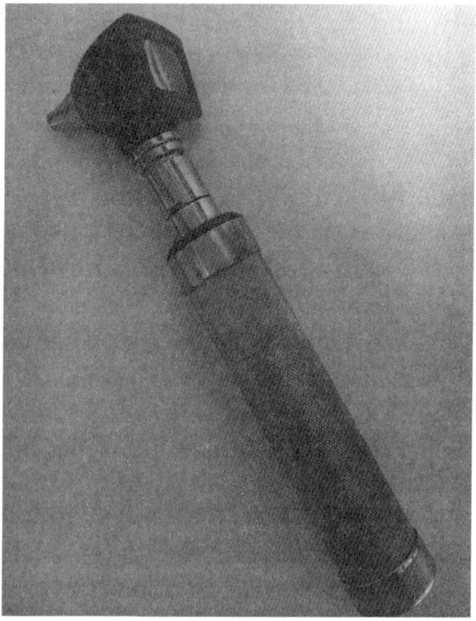

Figure 1–1. Standard otoscope.

- Incandescent: dull white color, less bright, hot
- Halogen: bluish-white color, bright, cool
- Xenon: very bright white light, warm
- LED (light-emitting diode): variety of colors, typically whitish-blue, brightest, cool

Power Source

There are several battery-power sources to choose from, each having unique characteristics.

- NiCad (nickel-cadmium): rechargeable, has memory effect (also known as voltage

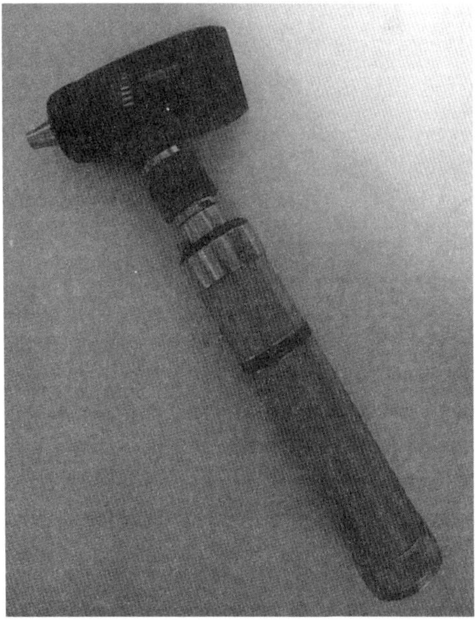

Figure 1–2. Wide-angle otoscope.

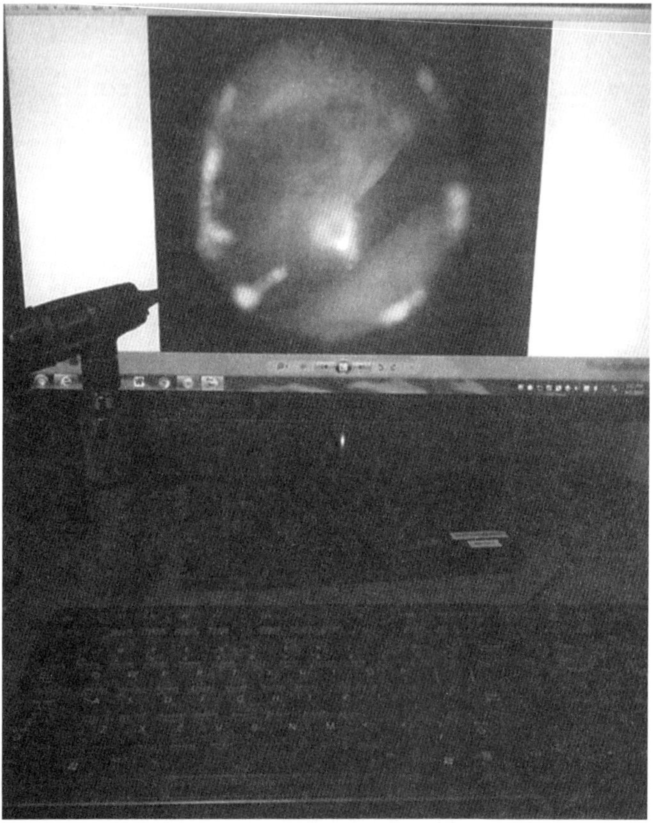

Figure 1–3. Video otoscope.

depression; improper charging can affect battery performance), medium-to-fast discharge rate, economical

- NiMH (nickel-metal hydride): rechargeable, no memory effect, medium to fast discharge rate, medium priced
- Li-ON (lithium-ion): rechargeable, no memory effect, slow discharge rate, higher initial cost

PROCEDURES

- Sit with your eyes slightly below patient ear-canal level and slightly behind the patient's shoulder. Examiner's stool and patient chair ergonomics should support appropriate viewing angles (Figure 1–4).
- Examine the pinna, surrounding skin, and tissue for any abnormalities, including discoloration and/or growths or surgical scars.

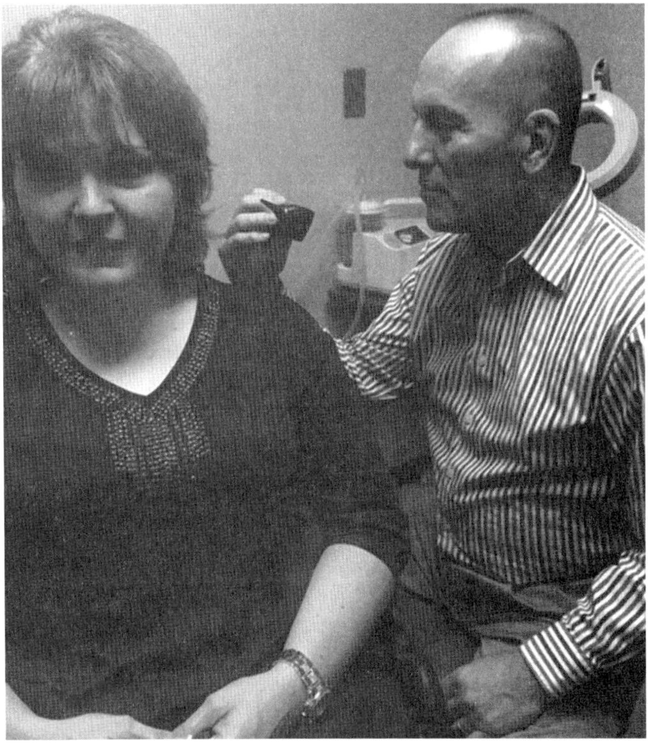

Figure 1–4. Examiner/patient positioning.

- Hold the otoscope near the otoscope head to minimize movement of the head/speculum. Your palm should be facing you as you hold the otoscope somewhat as you would hold a pencil, with the butt-end angled upward (Figure 1–5).
- For viewing the right ear canal hold the otoscope in your right hand. For viewing the left ear canal hold the otoscope in your left hand.
- Alternatively, you may hold the otoscope upright (head up). *Note:* This procedure is necessary with video otoscopes; a tilted otoscope is a tilted camera, which in turn results in a tilted image.
- Use your free hand to gently pull up and back on the adult patient's helix to aid in straightening out the ear canal. For children, the helix should be pulled down and back.

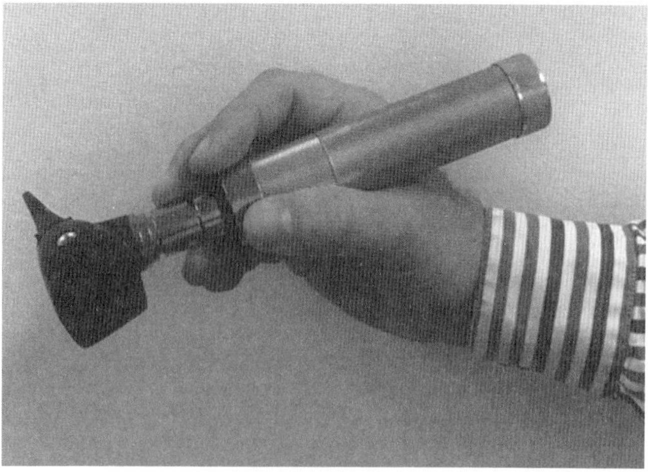

Figure 1–5. Holding the otoscope.

- Slowly insert the speculum into the ear canal making sure not to push too deep. Communicate with the patient about what to expect and allow the patient to provide feedback on comfort.
- Always brace (bridge) with one or two fingers on the patient's head, or by resting your wrist or arm on the patient's shoulder. With proper bridging, the otoscope will move when the patient moves, thus preventing the speculum from entering too far into the ear canal (Figure 1–6).
- Examine the ear canal and tympanic membrane/middle ear.

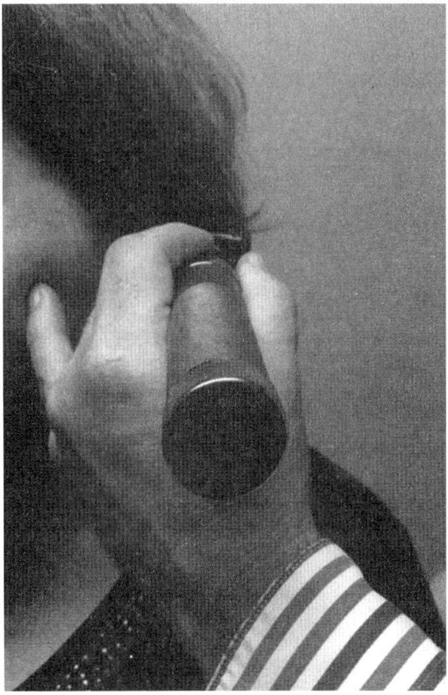

Figure 1–6. Bridging during otoscopy.

NORMAL PHYSICAL EXAMINATION AND OTOSCOPIC FINDINGS

Normal Pinna, Head, and Neck

- No signs of trauma or surgical scars
- No abrasions and lesions
- No malformations such as atresia, stenosis, tags, or abnormally positioned or angled pinna

Normal Ear Canal

- Minimal cerumen (cerumen amount can be graded none, minimal, moderate, or occluded)
- No abrasions and lesions
- No signs of infection, inflammation, otorrhea, or foreign bodies

Normal Tympanic Membrane and Middle Ear (Figure 1–7)

- Pinkish gray color and translucent
- Neither retracted nor bulging, resulting in a cone of light on the tympanic membrane in the anterior inferior quadrant
- Manubrium of the malleus pointing to 1:00 on the right tympanic membrane and 11:00 on the left tympanic membrane
- No signs of tympanic membrane infection, inflammation, otorrhea, damage
- No signs of neoplasm or effusion in the middle ear space

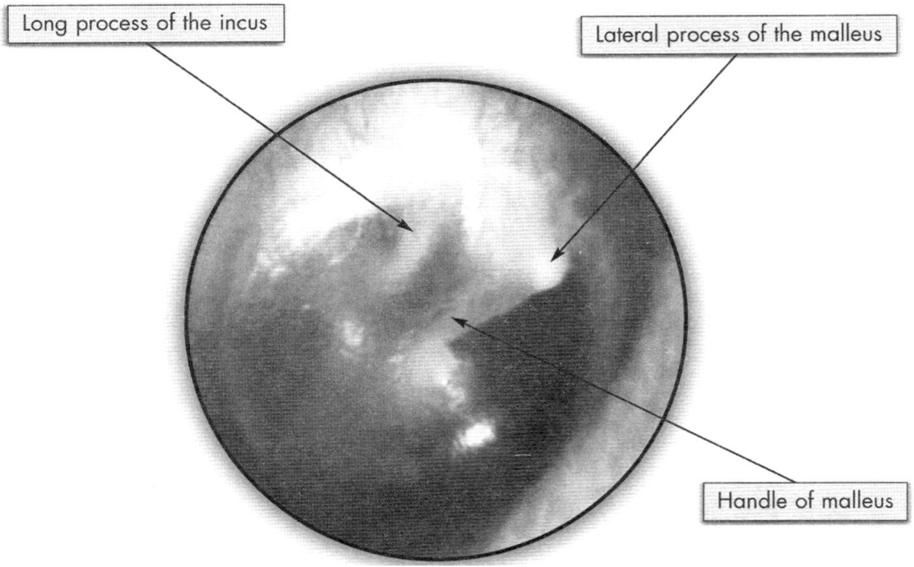

Figure 1–7. Normal tympanic membrane. From *Atlas of Otoscopy* (Page 7, Figure 1–6), by J. Touma and B. Touma, 2006, San Diego, CA: Plural Publishing, Inc. Reprinted with permission.

ABNORMAL OTOSCOPY EXAMPLES

- Figure 1–8 Exostosis: Benign boney growths in the ear canal
- Figure 1–9 Otomycosis: Fungal infection in the ear canal
- Figure 1–10 Serous otitis media: Middle ear effusion related to Eustachian tube dysfunction
- Figure 1–11 Acute otitis media: Rapid onset middle ear infection with a red (erythematic) bulging tympanic membrane

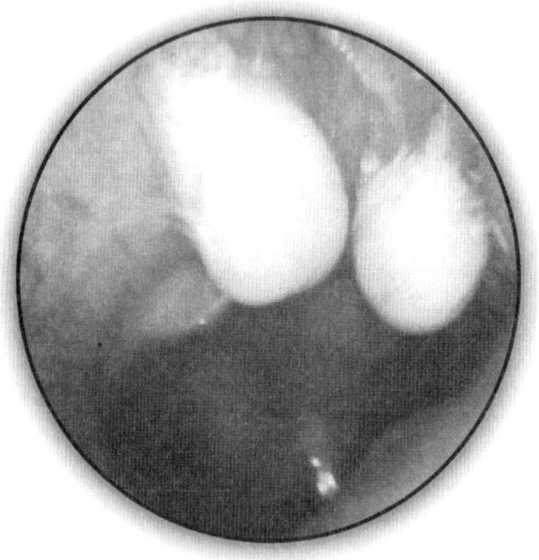

Figure 1–8. Exostosis. From *Atlas of Otoscopy* (Page 149, Figure 13–4), by J. Touma and B. Touma, 2006, San Diego, CA: Plural Publishing, Inc. Reprinted with permission.

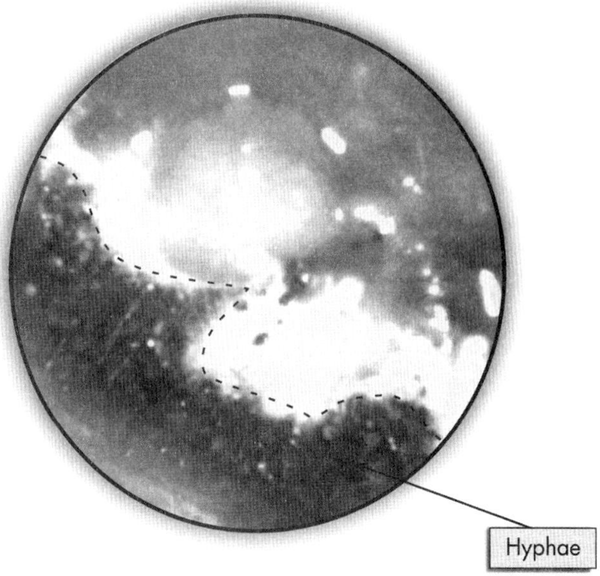

Figure 1–9. Otomycosis. From *Atlas of Otoscopy* (Page 158, Figure 15–1), by J. Touma and B. Touma, 2006, San Diego, CA: Plural Publishing, Inc. Reprinted with permission.

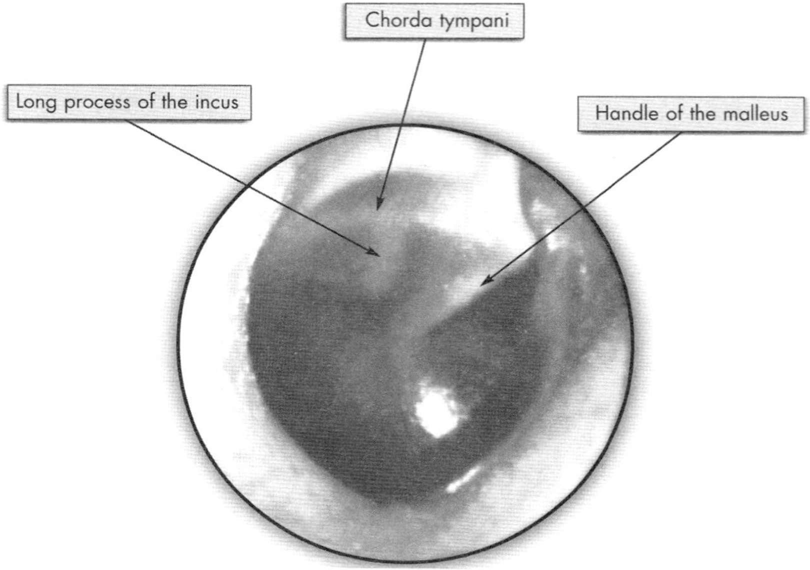

Figure 1–10. Serous otitis media. From *Atlas of Otoscopy* (Page 10, Figure 2–1), by J. Touma and B. Touma, 2006, San Diego, CA: Plural Publishing, Inc. Reprinted with permission.

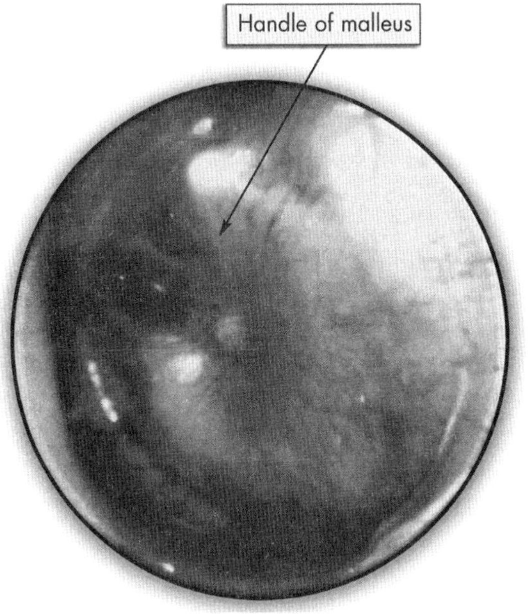

Figure 1–11. Acute otitis media. From *Atlas of Otoscopy* (Page 22, Figure 3–1), by J. Touma and B. Touma, 2006, San Diego, CA: Plural Publishing, Inc. Reprinted with permission.

- Figure 1–12 Ventilation (pressure equalization) Tubes: Tubes that aerate the middle ear as a treatment for Eustachian tube dysfunction
- Figure 1–13 Tympanosclerosis: Whitish tympanic membrane scar plaques
- Figure 1–14 Perforation: A hole in the tympanic membrane caused by infection, surgery, or trauma
- Figure 1–15 Cholesteatoma: Squamous epithelial cysts composed of keratin debris
- Figure 1–16 Glomus tumors: Benign, slow-growing, highly vascular neoplasms that arise from cells of the paraganglia

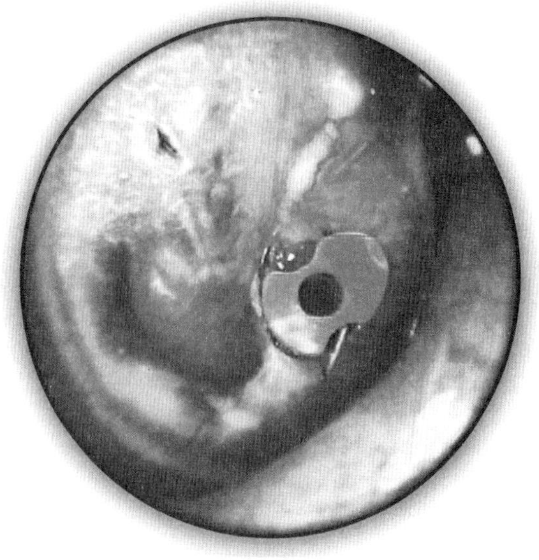

Figure 1–12. Ventilation tubes. From *Atlas of Otoscopy* (Page 34, Figure 4–1), by J. Touma and B. Touma, 2006, San Diego, CA: Plural Publishing, Inc. Reprinted with permission.

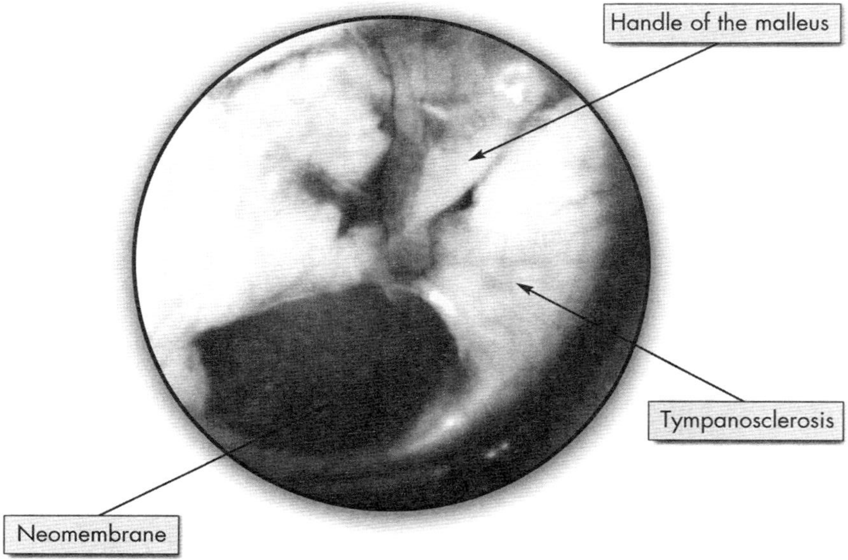

Figure 1–13. Tympanosclerosis. From *Atlas of Otoscopy* (Page 42, Figure 5–1), by J. Touma and B. Touma, 2006, San Diego, CA: Plural Publishing, Inc. Reprinted with permission.

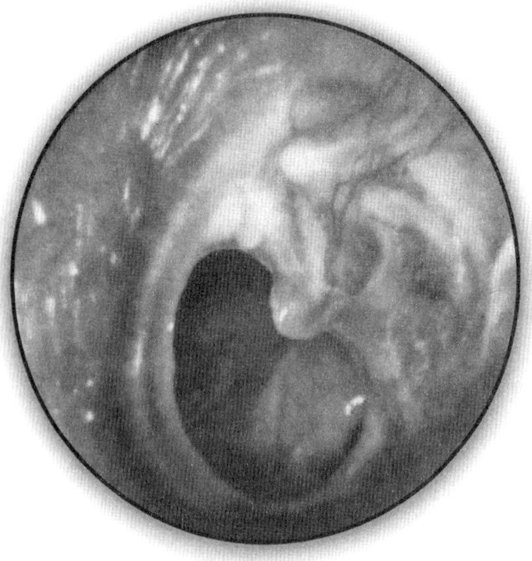

Figure 1–14. Perforation. From *Atlas of Otoscopy* (Page 68, Figure 7–5), by J. Touma and B. Touma, 2006, San Diego, CA: Plural Publishing, Inc. Reprinted with permission.

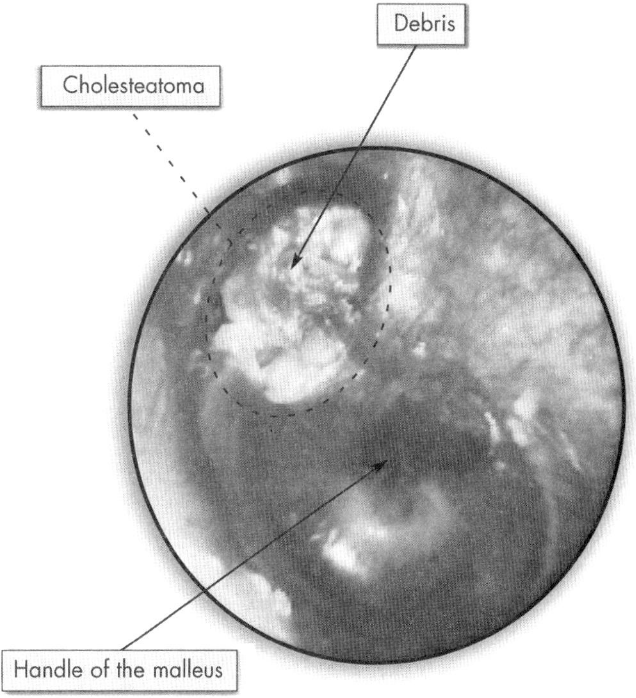

Figure 1–15. Cholesteatoma. From *Atlas of Otoscopy* (Page 109, Figure 10–10), by J. Touma and B. Touma, 2006, San Diego, CA: Plural Publishing, Inc. Reprinted with permission.

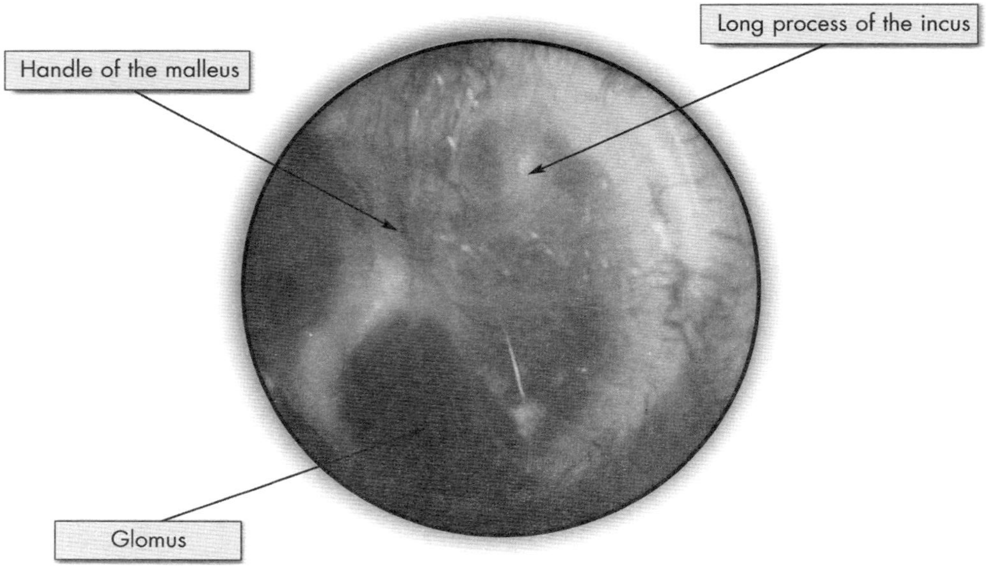

Figure 1–16. Glomus Tumor. From *Atlas of Otoscopy* (Page 152, Figure 14–1), by J. Touma and B. Touma, 2006, San Diego, CA: Plural Publishing, Inc. Reprinted with permission.

2

Pure-Tone Audiometry: Air Conduction

OVERVIEW OF PURE-TONE THRESHOLD EVALUATION

1. What is a pure-tone threshold
2. Why do we evaluate pure-tone thresholds
3. Procedures for evaluating air conduction pure-tone thresholds
4. Interpretation of pure-tone thresholds

WHAT IS A PURE-TONE THRESHOLD?

We measure hearing *sensitivity* as pure-tone "thresholds." We define threshold as the 50% correct detection point; this is an arbitrary, but agreed to, definition of threshold. With the measurement technique discussed below we approximate the 50% detection point with precision sufficient for routine clinical purposes.

WHY DO WE MEASURE AND EVALUATE PURE-TONE THRESHOLDS?

Basic pure-tone audiometry involves delivering pure-tones through either supra-aural or insert earphones, and is primarily a test of the peripheral hearing system. Precise site of lesion determination is difficult with air-conduction thresholds alone because a disorder anywhere in the peripheral system can result in abnormal thresholds. However, certain audiometric patterns can suggest a site of lesion and an etiology; for example, a 4000 Hz notch suggests noise exposure.

Importantly, we measure and evaluate pure-tone thresholds in order to determine if there is a loss of *hearing sensitivity* and to determine the *degree* of hearing sensitivity loss. This allows for preliminary gross estimation of handicap and/or prognosis.

INSTRUCTIONS

Instructions for pure-tone measurement are published by the American Speech-Language-Hearing Association (ASHA, 2005) and should include the following elements:

- Indicate the purpose of the test, that is, to find the faintest tone that can be heard.
- Indicate that the participant is to respond whenever the tone is heard, no matter how faint it may be.
- Describe the need to respond overtly as soon as the tone comes on and to respond overtly immediately when the tone goes off.

- Indicate that each ear is to be tested separately, with tones of different pitches.

Instruction Example

As per Martin (1998) the instructions to the patient are simple and direct.

> *I am going to place some earphones over your ears which will fit snugly. You will then hear some tones. Some of the tones will be loud, and others will be soft. Some will be in your left ear, and some will be in your right ear. Every time you hear a tone, raise your hand. Put your hand down when the tone stops. Remember to raise your hand, even if the tone is so soft you can barely hear it. Do you have any questions? (p. 23)*

Of course, these instructions must be altered when using insert earphones.

PATIENT RESPONSE OPTIONS

Patients may indicate when a tone is heard, for example, by raising a hand, raising a finger, pushing a response button, or saying "yes." The response mode should be decided with both efficiency and patient comfort and preference in mind.

PATIENT SEATING

The patient should be seated so that the audiologist's movements do not provide visual cues for tone presentations. At the same time, the audiologist should have sufficient view of the patient in order to monitor patient comfort and awareness. Seating the patient at a 90-degree angle to the audiologist should allow for both of these goals to be met.

CHOOSING THE TRANSDUCER FOR AIR-CONDUCTION PURE-TONE AUDIOMETRY

The two most common options for ear-specific air-conduction threshold measurement are supra-aural earphones and insert earphones.

Supra-Aural Earphones

Supra-aural earphones have the advantage of ease of use. However, supra-aural earphones have at least two disadvantages. The first is relatively low inter-aural crossover attenuation, which is important for masking. This is discussed in a later chapter. The second is that pressure from supra-aural earphones can collapse the cartilaginous portion of the ear canal, which would cause test results to mimic a conductive hearing loss.

Insert Earphones

There are several advantages for insert earphone use. Advantages include higher interaural crossover attenuation, which is important for masking, and elimination of the potential for collapsing ear canals. In addition, insert earphones are disposable and, therefore, hygienic. They are also better at reducing ambient noise during testing. However, a disadvantage is that insert earphone openings can become plugged by cerumen, which would cause test results to mimic a conductive hearing loss. Care should be taken to select the proper size to achieve, ideally, an insertion depth such that the outer edge is 2 to 3 mm within the ear canal.

Earphone Choice in Ears With Pressure Equalization Tubes, Perforated Tympanic Membranes, or Mastoid Bowls

Supra-aural earphones are recommended over insert earphones when patients have pressure equalization tubes, perforated tympanic membranes, or mastoid bowls from mastoidectomies. In ears with PE tubes, for example, insert earphone use can result in the overestimation of air-conduction hearing loss by as much as 14 dB at 250 Hz and as much as 10 dB at 500 Hz (Tokar-Prejna & Meinzen-Derr, 2006). Voss et al. (2000) showed similar results can be expected in ears with tympanic membrane perforations or mastoid bowls. Overestimation of air conduction hearing loss can result in misdiagnosis of conductive hearing loss or overestimation of the degree of conductive hearing loss. Voss et al. explained that the deep placement of insert earphones leaves a smaller residual ear canal volume than do supra-aural earphones. Therefore, the change in volume associated with the above conditions is proportionally greater with insert earphones. The proportionally greater volume change results in proportionally greater reductions in sound pressure level and thus poorer air-conduction thresholds.

TONE PRESENTATION TIPS

- Duration of pure-tone stimulus should be 1 to 2 seconds.
- Intervals between tone presentations must be varied so the patient cannot anticipate/guess when tones are presented.
- Start with a 30-dB (ASHA, 2005) tone to the better ear at 1000 Hz, or the right ear if no better ear is suspected. However, for returning patients, it is more time-efficient to present tones nearer their known thresholds.
- Pulsed tones are preferred by most patients (Burk & Wiley, 2004) and may be more readily identifiable to patients with tinnitus (Mineau & Schlauch, 1997), especially when testing at or near patients' tinnitus frequency.

THRESHOLD SEARCH PROCEDURE

Getting an Initial Response

- If your patient responds to a 30-dB tone, descend and present tones in 10-dB descending steps until the patient fails to respond to a tone.
- If the patient does not respond to a 30-dB tone, ascend and present a tone at 50 dB, and then in 10-dB ascending steps until a response is seen, or the limit of the audiometer is reached.

The Modified Hughson-Westlake Procedure

The Modified Hughson-Westlake procedure (Carhart & Jerger, 1959), commonly referred to as the "10 down 5 up" procedure, is the threshold measurement method of choice for routine audiologic practice. There are times when other techniques must be considered, such as with infants and children, and when pseudohypoacusis is suspected. Options are discussed later in this text.

- Whenever a patient responds to a tone, lower the intensity 10 dB and present another tone.
- Whenever a patient fails to respond to a tone, raise the intensity 5 dB and present another tone.
- Continue in this manner, keeping track of responses during ascending runs.

Threshold Definition

The American National Standards Institute (ANSI) (2004) recommends defining threshold as the lowest intensity level at which a patient responds to a minimum of two out of three tone presentations. This criterion, measured with the "10 down 5 up" technique, will allow us to approximate the 50% detection point with the precision sufficient for routine clinical purposes.

Alternative Threshold Definition

The ASHA (1978) recommended three responses at a single level. Harris (1979) and Tyler and Wood

(1980) found the ANSI and ASHA criteria yielded similar thresholds, but the ANSI criteria saved time.

Frequency Measurement Order

The ANSI (2004) recommended measuring pure-tone thresholds at the following frequencies and frequency order: 1000 Hz, 2000 Hz, 4000 Hz, 8000 Hz, re-measure at 1000 Hz, 500 Hz, and 250 Hz, and if a low-frequency hearing loss is present, 125 Hz. Test interoctaves (750 Hz, 1500 Hz, 3000 Hz, and/or 6000 Hz) when thresholds at flanking octaves differ by ≥20 dB. The ASHA (2005) recommended routine inclusion of 3000 Hz and 6000 Hz.

Note on re-measuring threshold at 1000 Hz: This is done as a response reliability check. The re-measured threshold should be within 5 dB of the originally measured threshold to be considered reliable. If the re-test threshold differs from the original by >5 dB, the lower of the two thresholds may be accepted, and at least one other test frequency should be retested. The audiologist must clearly document when thresholds are judged to be unreliable. Unreliable thresholds might be obtained for several reasons, including equipment malfunction and pseudohypoacusis. For details, see Chapter 18 on nonorganic hearing loss.

False Positives and False Negatives

Some patients will respond when no tone was heard (false positives) or fail to respond when tones were heard (false negatives). Subjects should be reinstructed and thresholds re-measured if a pattern of false positive or false negative responses are suspected.

Documenting Threshold

The appropriate unmasked air conduction threshold symbols are shown in Figure 2–1.

SIGNIFICANT THRESHOLD CHANGE CRITERIA

We often re-measure hearing thresholds to monitor for change. Significant change criteria proposed by ASHA (1994) include:

- 20 dB decrease at any one test frequency
- 10 dB decrease at any two or more adjacent frequencies
- Loss of response at three consecutive frequencies where responses were previously obtained

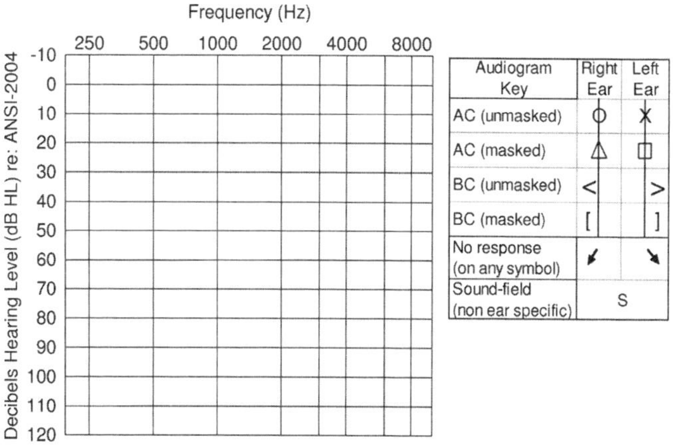

Figure 2–1. Audiogram and audiometric symbols. From *Audiology: Science to Practice* (2nd ed., p. 136, Figure 5–1), by S. Kramer, 2014, Plural Publishing, Inc. Reprinted with permission.

PURE-TONE AVERAGE (PTA)

PTA has several potential uses including:

- To help the audiologist summarize the degree of loss of sensitivity
- For use as a gross predictor or estimation of handicap and/or prognosis
- To compare to Speech Recognition Threshold (SRT) as a reliability check

Three-Frequency PTA

The most common PTA is a monaural three-frequency average of thresholds recorded at 500 Hz, 1000 Hz, and 2000 Hz. As Harrell (2002) states, "These [frequencies] are considered to represent the most important frequencies for understanding speech and therefore hold the most promise for estimating the degree of handicap that a particular hearing loss is likely to cause" (p. 81).

Two-Frequency PTA Option

The two-frequency PTA is calculated using the best two of three frequencies among 500, 1000, and 2000 Hz. This option is typically used to omit one threshold that is at least 20 dB poorer than the other two; such an outlier threshold might skew interpretation.

Less Commonly Used PTA Options

- Variable Pure-Tone Average (VPTA): worst three of 1000, 2000, 3000, and 4000 Hz (Clark, 1981)
- ASHA (1981): 1000, 2000, 3000, and 4000 Hz
- American Academy of Ophthalmology and Otolaryngology (AAOO) (1979): 500, 1000, 2000, 3000 Hz

Three Frequency PTA and Prediction of Handicap

Table 2–1 shows commonly used prediction guidelines for adults proposed by Goodman (1965), and guidelines for children proposed by Stewart and Downs (1984).

Table 2–1. Gross Handicap Predictions/Descriptors Based on the Three-Frequency Pure-Tone Average

ADULTS (Goodman, 1965)	*CHILDREN (Stewart & Downs, 1984)*
≤25 dB normal	<15 dB normal
	16–25 dB slight
26–40 dB mild	26–40 dB mild
41–55 dB moderate	41–55 dB moderate
56–70 dB moderately severe	56–70 dB moderately severe
71–90 dB severe	71–90 dB severe
91+ dB profound	91+ dB profound

Three-Frequency PTA Limitations

The PTA classifications are only *gross* hearing loss handicap predictors/descriptors because:

- Some PTA exclude frequencies 3000 Hz and above, which are important for speech understanding
- PTA does not take into account word recognition ability or auditory processing skills
- PTA ignores individual differences, including psychosocial factors

PERCENT HEARING LOSS FORMULAE

Percent Hearing Loss Formulae Generally Have Several Components

1. A PTA
2. A low fence dB level where hearing loss begins (typically 25 dB)
3. A high fence dB level where hearing loss is considered total
4. Hearing range: High fence–low fence
5. Percentage value assigned to each dB of hearing loss above the low fence: 100% ÷ the hearing range
6. A method of determining binaural percentage hearing loss

American Academy of Otolaryngology-Head and Neck Surgery (AAO-HNS) (1979) Formula

1. AAO-HNS PTA: 500 Hz, 1000 Hz, 2000 Hz, 3000 Hz
2. Low fence: 25 dB
3. High fence: 92 dB
4. Hearing range: 92 − 25 = 67 dB
5. Percentage assigned to each dB of hearing loss above the low fence: 100% ÷ 67 = 1.5%
6. Binaural percentage loss: (better ear percentage hearing loss times 5 + the poorer ear hearing loss) ÷ 6

Here is an example calculation for a patient with a right ear AAO-HNS PTA of 40 dB and a left ear AAO-HNS PTA of 50 dB:

- Assign 1.5% hearing loss for each dB above the low fence
    - Right ear 40 dB AAOO PTA − 25 dB low fence = 15 dB
    - 15 × 1.5 = 22.5% hearing loss
    - Left ear 50 dB AAOO PTA − 25 dB low fence = 25 dB
    - 25 × 1.5 = 37.5% hearing loss
- Binaural hearing loss:
    - (22.5% × 5) + 37.5% ÷ 6 = 25%

ASHA (1981) Formula

1. ASHA PTA: 1000 Hz, 2000 Hz, 3000 Hz, 4000 Hz
2. Low fence: 25 dB
3. High fence: 75 dB
4. Hearing range: 75 − 25 = 50 dB

5. Percentage assigned to each dB of hearing loss above the low fence 100% ÷ 50 = 2%.
6. Binaural percentage loss: (better ear percentage hearing loss times 5 + the poorer ear hearing loss) ÷ 6

Example calculation for a patient with a right ear ASHA PTA of 40 dB and a left ear ASHA PTA of 50 dB:

- Assign 2% hearing loss for each dB above the low fence
    - Right ear 40 dB ASHA PTA – 25 dB low fence = 15 dB
    - 15 × 2 = 30% hearing loss
    - Left ear 50 dB ASHA PTA – 25 dB low fence = 25 dB
    - 25 × 2 = 50% hearing loss
- Binaural hearing loss:
    - (30 × 5) + 50% ÷ 6 = 33.3%

Percent Hearing Loss Limitations

These formulae provide only a gross estimate of hearing impairment. John, Kreisman, and Pallett (2012) studied various PTA and percentage hearing loss formulae and found that they were significantly, but weakly correlated with self-reported hearing impairment. Nonetheless, percent hearing loss, as well as PTA, could be considered as potential counseling tools.

AGE-RELATED HEARING LOSS

Patients might be curious whether their hearing loss is consistent with age. This is a complicated judgment involving many factors. Nonetheless, this might be of value for counseling purposes. Table 2–2 shows presbycusis in males and females up to 60 years of age (American National Standards Institute, 1996).

AUDIOGRAM CONFIGURATION

Audiologists should note the audiogram configuration, as it might aid in diagnosis. Diagnostically significant audiogram configuration examples include:

Table 2–2. Presbycusis in Males and Females Screened for Noise Exposure (ANSI, 1996).

Males	*40 years*	*50 years*	*60 years*
500 Hz	11	14	18
1000 Hz	11	14	19
2000 Hz	15	21	29
3000 Hz	19	29	42
4000 Hz	23	37	55
6000 Hz	26	41	62
Females	***40 years***	***50 years***	***60 years***
500 Hz	11	14	18
1000 Hz	11	14	19
2000 Hz	13	18	25
3000 Hz	15	21	30
4000 Hz	17	25	35
6000 Hz	21	31	45

Note. The data above is in dB HL. Only 10% of people are worse than levels shown.

3000, 4000, or 6000 Hz noise-induced hearing loss notches; high-frequency sensory presbycusis hearing losses; and low-frequency hearing losses for Ménière's disease. Table 2–3 shows the audiogram descriptors the authors recommend.

ASYMMETRY

Certain disorders, such as acoustic neuromas and Meniere's disease, manifest as asymmetric hearing sensitivity. Therefore, audiologists must have crite-

Table 2–3. Audiogram Configuration Descriptors

Flat	Thresholds are within 20 dB of each other across the frequency range
Rising	Thresholds for low frequencies are at least 20 dB poorer than for high frequencies
Sloping	Thresholds for high frequencies are at least 20 dB poorer than for low frequencies
Low frequency	Hearing loss is restricted to the low frequency region of the audiogram
High frequency	Hearing loss is restricted to the high frequency region of the audiogram
Precipitously sloping	Steeply sloping high frequency hearing loss of at least 20 dB per octave
Trough or cookie bite	Thresholds for mid frequencies are at least 20 dB poorer than thresholds at 250 or 8000 Hz
Notched	Threshold at one frequency at least 10 dB poorer than adjacent frequencies

Note. The first five are given by Stach (1998, page 107) and the last two are used in our clinic.

ria to serve as tools for determination of significant asymmetry. Several asymmetry criteria have been proposed and are discussed further in the medical referral chapter in this text. We will mention two options here. The first are the AAO PTA (1993, 1994) asymmetry criteria: a difference of >15 dB between the AAO PTA of the right and left ears. The AAO PTA frequencies are 500 Hz, 1000 Hz, 2000 Hz, and 3000 Hz. The second criteria offered here are the interaural difference at two adjacent frequencies of 15 dB in unilateral hearing loss and 20 dB in bilateral asymmetric loss (Obholzer, Rea, & Harcourt, 2004). These latter criteria offer sensitivity (97%) higher and specificity (49%) lower than the AAO-HNS criteria.

PEDIATRIC PURE-TONE THRESHOLD EVALUATION

A full discussion of pediatric threshold measurement is beyond the scope of this text; a brief overview follows. There are three generally accepted approaches to pediatric threshold evaluation: behavioral response audiometry (BOA), visually reinforced audiometry (VRA), and play audiometry. The developmental age of the patient often dictates the procedure first attempted (Table 2–4).

Behavioral Response Audiometry (BOA)

BOA might be best for patients of developmental age 1 to 4 months. The infant is placed in an appropriate seat, or on the mothers lap, and stimuli are presented through speakers or under earphones. The audiologist watches for patient responses in the

Table 2–4. Pediatric Evaluation Table for Behavioral Observation Audiometry (BOA), Visually Reinforced Audiometry (VRA), and Play Audiometry

	BOA	***VRA***	***Play Audiometry***
Age	1 to 4 months	4 months to 2 years	2 to 5 years
Stimuli	Running speech or warbled tones	Running speech or warbled tones	Pure-tones, spondee threshold search
Transducer	Speakers or earphones	Speakers or earphones	Earphones
Response mode	Change in demeanor or behavior	Localize/ lateralize	Behavioral response such as placing a block in a bucket
Test result	Minimum response level	Minimum response level	Threshold
Approximate normal for speech (Northern & Downs, 2002)	45 dB MRL for running speech	20 dB MRL for running speech at 4 to 7 months improving to approximately 5 dB at 2 years	0–15 dB spondee thresholds
Approximate normal for tones (Northern & Downs, 2002)	70 dB MRL for tones	50 dB MRL for tones at 4 to 7 months improving to approximately 25 dB at 2 years	0–15 dB pure-tone thresholds

form of changes in demeanor, behavior, or mood. The lowest intensity at which a response is obtained is called the minimum response level (MRL). The MRL will be greater than true threshold. Norms are given in Table 2–4.

Visually Reinforced Audiometry (VRA)

VRA might be best for patients of developmental age 4 months to 2 years. The child is typically seated between two speakers, each at a 45-degree angle, or under earphones. The audiologist watches for patient responses. In the sound field, the response would be head turning to the right or left speaker in response to the stimuli presented. A VRA requires a conditioning phase during which stimuli and visual reward (e.g., a lighted toy) are presented simultaneously. During the testing phase, the reward is given only after a correct response. The lowest intensity at which a response is obtained is called the minimum response level (MRL). The MRL will be greater than true threshold. Norms are given in Table 2–4.

Play Audiometry

Play audiometry might be best for patients 2 years or older. The child listens under earphones and gives a behavioral response when tones are heard. The behavioral response is made interesting, such as dropping a block into a bucket. Play audiometry requires a conditioning phase during which the task is taught, followed by the testing phase. The lowest intensity at which a response is obtained is considered true threshold.

REFERENCES

American Academy of Ophthalmology and Otolaryngology Committee on Hearing and Equilibrium and the American Council of Otolaryngology Committee on the Medical Aspects of Noise. (1979). Guide for the evaluation of hearing handicap. *Journal of the American Medical Association*, *241*, 2055–2059.

American Academy Otolaryngology and American Council of Otolaryngology. (1979). Guide for the evaluation of hearing handicap. *Journal of the American Medical Association*, *241*, 2056–2079.

American Academy of Otolaryngology–Head and Neck Surgery. (1993). *Bulletin*, 16–17.

American Academy of Otolaryngology–Head and Neck Surgery. (1994). *Bulletin*, 26–28.

American National Standards Institute. (1996). *Determination of noise exposure and estimation of noise induced hearing impairment*. (ANSI S3.44-1996). New York, NY: Acoustical Society of America.

American National Standards Institute. (2004). *Methods for manual pure-tone threshold audiometry*. (ANSI S3.21-2004). New York, NY: Author.

American Speech-Language-Hearing Association. (1978). Guidelines for manual pure-tone threshold audiometry. *ASHA*, *20*, 297–301.

American Speech-Language-Hearing Association. (1981). *On the definition of hearing handicap*. Retrieved from http:www.asha.org/policy

American Speech-Language-Hearing Association. (1994). Guidelines for the audiologic management of individuals receiving cochleotoxic drug therapy. *ASHA*, *36*, 11–19.

American Speech-Language-Hearing Association. (2005). *Guidelines for manual pure-tone threshold audiometry*. Retrieved from http:www.asha.org/policy

Burk, M. H., & Wiley, T. L. (2004). Continuous versus pulsed tones in audiometry. *American Journal of Audiology*, *13*, 54–61.

Carhart, R., & Jerger, J. F. (1959). Preferred method for clinical determination of pure-tone thresholds. *Journal of Speech and Hearing Disorders*, *24*, 330–345.

Clark, J. G. (1981). Uses and abuses of hearing loss clarification. *ASHA*, *23*, 493–500.

Goodman, A. (1965). Reference zero levels for pure-tone audiometer. *ASHA*, *7*, 262–263.

Harris, J. D. (1979). Optimum thrilled crossings and time window validation in threshold pure-tone audiometry. *Journal of the Acoustical Society of America*, *66*, 1545–1547.

Harrell, R. W. (2002). Puretone evaluation. In J. Katz (Ed.), *Handbook of clinical audiology* (5th ed., p. 81). Baltimore, MD: Lippincott Williams & Wilkins.

John, A. B., Kreisman, B. M., & Pallett, S. (2012). Validity of hearing impairment calculation methods for prediction of self-reported hearing handicap. *Noise and Health*, *14* (56), 13–20.

Martin, F. N. (1998). *Exercises in audiometry: A laboratory manual* (p. 23). Boston, MA: Allyn & Bacon.

Mineau, S. M., & Schlauch, R. S. (1997). Threshold measurement for patients with tinnitus: Pulsed or continuous tones. *American Journal of Audiology*, *6*, 52–56.

Northern, J. L., & Downs, M. P. (2002). *Hearing in children* (5th ed.). Baltimore, MD: Lippincott Williams & Wilkins.

Obholzer, R. J., Rea, P. A., & Harcourt, J. P. (2004). Magnetic resonance imaging screening for vestibular schwannoma: Analysis of published protocols. *Journal of Laryngology & Otology*, *118*, 329–332. http://dx.doi.org/10.1258/002221504323086480

Stach, B.A. (1998). *Clinical audiology: An introduction*. San Diego, CA: Singular.

Stewart, J. M., & Downs, M. P. (1984). Medical management of the hearing-handicapped child. In J. L. Northern (Ed.), *Hearing disorders* (2nd ed., pp. 267–278). Boston, MA: Little, Brown.

Tokar-Prejna, S., & Meinzen-Derr, J. (2006). Relationship between transducer type and low-frequency hearing loss for patients with ventilation tubes. *International Journal of Pediatric Otolaryngology*, *70*, 1063–1067.

Tyler, R. S., & Wood, E. J. (1980). A comparison of manual methods for measuring hearing levels. *International Society of Audiology*, *19*, 316–329.

Voss, S. E., Rosowski, J. J., Merchant, S. N., Thornton, A. R., Shera, C. A., & Peake, W. T. (2000). Middle ear pathology can affect the ear-canal sound pressure generated by audiologic earphones. *Ear and Hearing*, *21*(4), 265–274.

3

Pure-Tone Audiometry: Bone Conduction

THERE ARE SEVERAL ANATOMICAL CONTRIBUTORS TO BONE CONDUCTION HEARING

- The outer ear contributes, at times, to bone conduction hearing.
- The middle ear contributes to bone conduction hearing.
- The inner ear contributes to bone conduction hearing.
- Non-osseous skull contents contribute, at times, to bone conduction hearing.

Regardless of anatomical contributor, the end results are traveling waves and sensorineural stimulation in the same manner as for air conduction.

Outer Ear Component of Bone Conduction

Bone-conducted tones vibrate the skull, including the walls of the ear canal. In turn, air molecules in the ear canal are set into vibration; thus a sound wave results and hearing is possible by the exploitation of the air conduction pathway (Stenfelt & Goode, 2005; Tonndorf, 1968). This so-called "osseotympanic" bone conduction may play a small role in the normal unoccluded ear canal. However, low-frequency *bone conduction* energy is trapped when the outer ear is occluded, and this enhances bone conduction hearing in the lower audiometric test frequencies (Stenfelt & Goode, 2005).

Middle Ear Component of Bone Conduction

Bone-conducted tones vibrate the skull and also the ossicular chain. The ossicular chain is not rigidly attached to the middle ear walls; instead, it is, suspended by ligaments, tendons, and attachment to the tympanic and oval window membranes. Therefore, the ossicles are free to move out of phase with the skull vibrations because of inertia, much as coffee would lag and spill from a cup moved precipitously. Thus, middle ear ossicles vibrate out of phase with the skull in like manner, as during air conduction hearing (Barany, 1938; Steiger, 2015).

The middle ear component typically adds to bone conduction hearing at and around 2000 Hz, the approximate resonant frequency of the middle ear (Carhart, 1950). Alteration of the middle ear bone conduction component therefore can lower (make worse) 2000 Hz bone conduction thresholds. This lowering of bone conduction thresholds should not be diagnosed as a sensorineural hearing loss; it is a pseudo-sensorineural hearing loss.

Inner Ear Component of Bone Conduction

The cochlear fluids and membranes are free to move out of phase with bone vibrator-induced skull compressions and distortions, and they will do so, again, much as coffee would lag and spill from a cup moved precipitously, resulting in traveling waves.

Non-Osseous Skull Content Bone Conduction

Bone conduction energy can travel in non-osseous skull contents such as the brain, membranes, and fluids, and reach the cochlea through the cochlear and/or vestibular aqueducts. Non-osseous skull content bone conduction normally plays little if any role. (Stenfelt & Goode, 2005). In certain disorders, as discussed below, this bone conduction mode is enhanced.

BONE VIBRATOR

Bone vibrators are transducers whose diaphragms are encased in plastic. A metal headband holds the circular plastic surface of the bone vibrator in contact with the patient's skull, typically at the better ear mastoid, or the right mastoid if no better ear is known or suspected.

PROCEDURES

The procedures for measuring bone conduction thresholds are similar to those discussed for air conduction audiometry, with the exception of frequencies tested: 1000 Hz, 2000 Hz, and 4000 Hz, an optional retest of 1000 Hz (if poor reliability is suspected), 500 Hz and 250 Hz (ASHA, 1990). Use appropriate, unmasked threshold symbols shown in Figure 2–1. *Note.* Audiometric zero, as established by ANSI (2004), assumes contralateral ear masking. The authors' experience is that unmasked bone conduction thresholds are often inaccurate at 250 Hz and 4000 Hz. For unmasked bone conduction threshold evaluation, we, therefore, recommend testing at 500, 1000, and 2000 Hz. Should air-bone threshold gaps be measured and masking initiated, we then recommend expanding testing to include 250 Hz and 4000 Hz.

NORMAL HEARING SENSITIVITY

For patients with normal hearing, air and bone conduction thresholds are within normal limits and within +/− 10 dB of one another. Energy reaches the cochlea unimpeded by both the air conduction pathway and the bone conduction pathways, mainly the middle- and inner-ear bone conduction pathways. Sensory/neural functioning is normal.

SENSORY/NEURAL HEARING LOSS

For patients with sensory/neural hearing, air and bone conduction thresholds are within +/− 10 dB of one another, but neither is within normal limits. Energy reaches the cochlea unimpeded by both the air conduction pathway and the bone conduction pathways, mainly the middle and inner ear bone conduction pathways. However, sensory/neural functioning is not normal, worsening both air and bone conduction thresholds.

CONDUCTIVE HEARING LOSS FROM OUTER EAR OCCLUSION AND AIR-BONE GAPS OF OUTER EAR ORIGIN

For patients with conductive hearing loss from outer ear occlusions, air conduction thresholds are >10 dB poorer than normal bone conduction thresholds; the so-called air-bone gap. Energy reaches the cochlea unimpeded by the bone conduction pathways, mainly the middle and inner ear pathways. Because sensory/neural functioning is normal, bone conduction thresholds are normal. In contrast, the occlusion impedes the air conduction pathway, thus air conduction thresholds are >10 dB poorer than bone conduction thresholds. An occlusion effect might also manifest: An outer ear occlusion might trap outer-ear component bone conducted energy that would normally exit the ear canal. In such cases, low frequency bone conduction thresholds might be better (lower) than normal or expected.

CONDUCTIVE HEARING LOSS FROM MIDDLE EAR DISORDER AND AIR-BONE GAPS OF MIDDLE EAR ORIGIN

Air conduction thresholds are >10 dB poorer than normal bone conduction thresholds: the so-called air-bone gap. Energy reaches the cochlea unimpeded by the bone conduction pathways, mainly the middle and inner ear pathways. Because sensory/neural functioning is normal, bone conduction thresholds are normal. In contrast, the middle ear disorder impedes the air conduction pathway, thus air conduction thresholds are >10 dB poorer than bone conduction thresholds.

Middle ear disorders, such as stapedial fixation from otosclerosis, might disrupt middle ear bone conduction and thus alter middle ear resonance. This typically manifests as a loss of the normal 2000 Hz middle ear resonance. This results in a worsening of bone conduction hearing at 2000 Hz, the so-called Carhart notch. Audiologists typically use bone conduction thresholds to infer sensory/neural reserve, but they would be unwise to do so at 2000 Hz in cases of ossicular fixation. Instead, that loss of bone-conduction hearing at 2000 Hz can be called a pseudo-sensory/neural hearing loss (Hall & Croutch, 2008; Tonndorf, 1968).

Similarly, small pseudo-sensory/neural hearing loss has been reported in otitis media and glue ear. Even cerumen impaction can cause pseudo-sensory/neural hearing loss if it is impinging ("loading") on the tympanic membrane. The bone conduction notch for otitis media or glue ear has been reported at 1000 Hz, less often at 2000 Hz (Carhart, 1950; Hall & Croutch, 2008; Kumar, Maheshwar, Mahendran, Oluwasamni & Clayton, 2003; Yasan, 2007).

MIXED CONDUCTIVE AND SENSORY/NEURAL HEARING LOSS

When there is a sensory/neural disorder, neither air conduction thresholds nor bone conduction thresholds are within normal limits. However, air conduction thresholds are >10 dB worse than normal bone conduction thresholds because of outer or middle ear disorder: the so-called air-bone gap.

NOTE ON THE MAXIMUM AIR-BONE GAP

The maximum air-bone threshold gap is approximately 60 dB for adults because higher intensity air-conducted stimuli will cause the skull to vibrate (Bekesy, 1960). Therefore, air conducted stimuli presented > 60 dB are likely to be heard, albeit by bone conduction.

SUPERIOR SEMICIRCULAR CANAL DEHISCENCE (SSCD) AND AIR-BONE GAPS OF INNER EAR ORIGIN

With SSCD, energy reaches the cochlea unimpeded by both the air conduction pathway and the middle and inner ear bone conduction pathways. However, air conduction thresholds are poorer than normal, or expected, because air conducted energy is shunted away from the cochlea through the superior semicircular canal dehiscence (Steiger, 2015); a thinning of bone effectively forms a third inner-ear window (the first two being the oval and round windows). This typically manifests as hearing loss in the lower test frequencies (Merchant, Rosowski, & McKenna, 2007).

At the same time, bone conduction thresholds might be better than air conduction thresholds. With SSCD, the dehiscence opens a non-osseous bone conduction route passing more bone-conducted energy than normal to sensory/neural structures. In fact, in some cases, bone conduction thresholds might be normal or even better than expected (Attias et al., 2012; Chien, Janky, Minor, & Carey, 2012; Merchant et al., 2007).

Avoiding Misdiagnosis of Conductive Hearing Loss

Air-bone gaps of inner ear origin should not be called conductive hearing loss. The term conductive hearing loss should be reserved for outer ear occlusions, or middle ear disorders in which bone conducted energy is impeded. In patients with SSCD, bone conducted energy is not impeded, and the site of lesion is the superior semicircular canal.

Avoiding Misdiagnosis of Sensory/Neural Hearing Loss

Though the site of lesion with SSCD is in the inner ear, the hearing loss might not reflect damage to hair cells and/or neurons. Instead, at least some of the hearing loss can be called pseudo-sensory/neural.

LARGE (OR ENLARGED) VESTIBULAR AQUEDUCTS (LVA), SENSORY/NEURAL HEARING LOSS, AND AIR-BONE GAPS OF INNER EAR ORIGIN

With LVA, energy reaches the cochlea unimpeded by both the air conduction pathway and the middle and inner ear bone conduction pathways. Sensory/

neural structures (hair cells and neurons) may be disordered from trauma to hair cells by endolymph pressure through the endolymphatic duct and sac, or by endolymph electrolyte content that is harmful to the hair cells or stria vascularis (Campbell, Adunka, Zhou, Qaqish, & Buchman, 2011; Jackler & De La Cruz, 1989; Levinson, Parisier, Jacobs, & Edelstein, 1989).

However, air conduction thresholds might be further worsened by a shunting of air-conducted energy away from the cochlea through the LVA. At the same time, bone conduction thresholds might be better than expected because the LVA opens a non-osseous bone conduction route, passing more bone-conducted energy than normal to sensory/neural structures (Attias et al. 2102; Merchant et al., 2007).

Avoiding Misdiagnosis of Conductive Component to the Hearing Loss

Air-bone gaps of inner ear origin should not be called conductive hearing loss. The term conductive hearing loss should be reserved for outer ear occlusions, or middle ear disorders in which bone conducted energy is not impeded. In patients with LVA, bone conducted thresholds might be enhanced, but the site of lesion is the vestibular aqueduct.

Avoiding Misdiagnosis of Sensory/Neural Hearing Loss

Though the site of lesion with LVA is in the inner ear, not all of the hearing loss is caused by hair cell and neural disorder. Some of the hearing loss is due to energy being shunted away through the LVA.

Therefore, at least some of the hearing loss might be pseudo-sensory/neural.

INTRACRANIAL HYPERTENSION (IH)

Similar to sensory/neural hearing loss, air and bone conduction thresholds are within +/− 10 dB of one another, but neither is within normal limits. However, patients might present with pseudo-sensory/neural hearing loss resulting not from hair cell or neural disorder, but instead from one of two possible causes. The first is elevated cochlear fluid pressure passing into the cochlea through the vestibular or cochlear aqueducts. The cochlear fluid pressure could stiffen cochlear membranes and inhibit traveling waves (Sismanis, 1987). The second possible cause is masking of hearing by the pulsatile tinnitus, also passing through the vestibular or cochlear aqueducts (Rudnick & Sismanis, 2005; Steiger et al., 2007). Intracranial hypertension has been associated with syringohydromyelia, Chiari malformations, trauma, tumors, arachnoiditis, subarachnoid hemorrhages, meningitis, and multiple sclerosis.

VIBROTACTILE BONE-CONDUCTION RESPONSES

Patients might feel bone conductor diaphragm vibrations, especially at high intensities and at lower test frequencies. Therefore, audiologists should be vigilant, especially when low-frequency bone-conduction thresholds are inconsistent with other audiometric findings or history. In such cases, audiologists should ask such patients whether they heard or felt the tones. Failure to identify vibrotactile bone conduction responses could result in one of two misdiagnoses (Nober, 1964):

1. Vibrotactile bone conduction responses could be better than air conduction thresholds suggesting mixed hearing loss that might not exist.
2. Vibrotactile bone conduction responses might occur in a deaf patient, suggesting hearing when there was none.

THRESHOLD ACCURACY AND THE AIR-BONE GAP

Patient response variability can result in either underestimated or exaggerated air-bone threshold gaps, or even bone-air threshold gaps (Margolis, 2008; Studebaker, 1967).

TUNING FORK TESTS

Weber Tuning Fork Test Procedure and Stimuli

Conduct this test on listeners with asymmetrical hearing loss. Use 256 and/or 512 Hz tuning forks or 250 and/or 500 Hz through the bone vibrator at approximately 40 dB HL. The tuning fork or bone vibrator is applied to the forehead at the midline, and the patient is asked to indicate if the tone is heard in their right ear, left ear, or midline (can't localize).

Weber Results

- Listeners with asymmetrical conductive hearing loss might hear bone-conducted tones as louder in the impaired ear due to the occlusion effect.
- Listeners with asymmetrical sensory/neural hearing loss might hear bone-conducted tones as softer in the impaired ear due to the sensorineural disorder.

The Rinne Tuning Fork Test Procedure and Stimuli

Conduct this test on any listeners with hearing loss. Use 256 and/or 512 Hz tuning forks or 250 and/or 500 Hz through the bone vibrator at approximately 40 dB HL. The tuning fork or bone vibrator is alternately applied to the mastoid of the impaired ear (bone conduction hearing) and positioned in front of the impaired ear (air conduction hearing); the patient judges which is louder.

Rinne Results

- Negative Rinne: Listeners with conductive hearing loss might hear louder by bone conduction in the ear being tested due to the occlusion effect, and because an occlusive disorder will attenuate air-conducted tones.
- False negative Rinne: Listeners with unilateral sensory/neural hearing loss might hear louder by bone conduction because they hear it in their normal ear, the ear not being tested, misleading the clinician to assume a negative Rinne.

- Positive Rinne: Listeners with sensory/neural hearing loss might hear louder by air conduction in the ear being tested because it's easier to vibrate air molecules than bone.

REFERENCES

American Speech-Language-Hearing Association. (1990). Guidelines for audiometric symbols. *ASHA*, *32*, 25–30.

American National Standards Institute. (2004). *Methods for manual pure-tone threshold audiometry.* (ANSI S3.21-2004). New York, NY: Author.

Attias, J., Ulanovski, D., Shemesh, R., Kornreich, L., Nageris, B., Preis, . . . Raveh, E. (2012). Air-bone gap component of inner-ear origin in audiograms of cochlear implant candidates. *Otology & Neurotology*, *33*, 512–517.

Barany, E. (1938). A contribution to the physiology of bone conduction. *Acta Otolaryngologica*, *26*, 1–223. Retrieved from http://www.tandfonline.com/toc/ioto20/current

Bekesy, G. (1960). *Experiments in hearing.* New York, NY: McGraw-Hill.

Campbell, A. P., Adunka, O. F., Zhou, B., Qaqish, B. F., & Buchman, C. A. (2011). Large vestibular aqueduct syndrome. *Laryngoscope*, *121*, 352–357.

Carhart, R. (1950). Clinical application of bone conduction audiometry. *Archives of Otolaryngology*, *51*, 798–808.

Chien, W. W., Janky, K., Minor, L. B., & Carey, J. P. (2012). Superior semicircular canal dehiscence size: Multivariate assessment of clinical impact. *Otology & Neurotology*, *33*, 810–815.

Hall, C. M., & Croutch, C. (2008) Pseudosensory-neural hearing loss. *Hearing Review*, *16*(1), 18–22.

Jackler, R. K., & De La Cruz, A. (1989) The large vestibular aqueduct syndrome. *Laryngoscope*, *99*(12), 1238-1243.

Kumar, M., Maheshwar, A., Mahendran, S., Oluwasamni, A., & Clayton, M. I. (2003). Could the presence of a

Carhart notch predict the presence of glue at myringotomy? *Clinical Otolaryngology, 28*(3), 183–186.

Levinson, M. J., Parisier, S. C., Jacobs, M., & Edelstein, D. R. (1989). The large vestibular aqueduct syndrome in children: A review of 12 cases and the description of a new clinical entity. *Advances in Otorhinolaryngology, 115*, 54–58.

Margolis, R.H. (2008). The vanishing air-bone gap: Audiology's dirty little secret. *Audiology Online*. Retrieved from http://www.audiologyonline.com/articles/vanishing-air-bone-gap-audiology-901&referer=www.clickfind.com.au

Merchant, S. N., Rosowski, J. J., & McKenna, M. J. (2007). Superior semicircular canal dehiscence mimicking otosclerotic hearing loss. *Advances in Otorhinolaryngology, 65*, 137–145.

Nober, E. H. (1964). Pseudoauditory bone conduction thresholds. *Journal of Speech and Hearing Disorders, 29*, 469–476.

Rudnick, E., & Sismanis, A. (2005). Pulsatile tinnitus and spontaneous cerebrospinal fluid rhinorrhea: Indicators of benign intracranial hypertension syndrome. *Otology & Neurotology, 26*(2), 166–168.

Sismanis, A. (1987). Otologic manifestations of benign intracranial hypertension syndrome: Diagnosis and management. *Laryngoscope, 97*, 1–17. http://dx.doi.org/10.1288/00005537-198708001-00001

Steiger, J. R. (2015). Bone conduction evaluation. In J. Katz, M. Chasin, K. English, L. Hood, & K. Tillery (Eds.), *Handbook of clinical audiology* (7th ed., pp. 49–58). Philadelphia, PA: Wolters Kluwer.

Steiger, J. R., Saccone, P., & Watson, K. N. (2007). Assessment of objective pulsatile tinnitus in a patient with syringohydromyelia. *Journal of American Academy of Audiology, 18*(3), 197–206.

Stenfelt, S. & Goode, R. L. (2005). Bone-conducted sound: Physiological and clinical aspects. *Otology & Neurotology, 26*, 1245–1261.

Studebaker, G. A. (1967). Clinical masking of the non-test ear. *Journal of Speech and Hearing Disorders*, *32*, 360–371.

Tonndorf, J. (1968). A new concept of bone conduction. *Archives of Otolaryngology*, *87*, 49–54.

Yasan, H. (2007). Predictive role of Carhart's notch in pre-operative assessment for middle-ear surgery. *Journal of Laryngology & Otology*, *121*, 219–221.

4

Pure-Tone Air-Conduction Masking

THE PROBLEM

A tone presented through an earphone to the test ear (TE) can "crossover" and be heard in the non-test ear (NTE). Air-conducted (AC) sound waves of sufficient intensity vibrate the cartilaginous and bony external auditory meatus of the test ear, and sound waves travel by bone conduction (BC) to both the test ear and non-test ear cochlea.

MASKING

We deliver noise through an earphone to the NTE to "mask" it, that is, to elevate the NTE threshold so that the patient will not be able to hear tones that have crossed over to it. For example, masking delivered 30 dB above the NTE AC threshold will elevate the NTE AC threshold *and* NTE BC threshold by 30 dB. With sufficient masking, the NTE threshold will be elevated to a level rendering it unable to hear test tones.

WHEN TO MASK

Insert Earphones

When sound crosses from the TE to the NTE it will be attenuated by the skull and skull contents. The amount of attenuation, called interaural attenuation (IA), is frequency-dependent. Yacullo (2009) concluded we should assume IA is 75 dB for frequencies ≤1000 Hz but only 50 dB for frequencies >1000 Hz. Therefore one can determine the need for masking with insert earphones with the following two rules:

- For test frequencies 250 Hz through 1000 Hz: Mask the NTE when the TE AC threshold is more than 75 dB greater than the NTE BC threshold.
- For test frequencies 2000 Hz through 8000 Hz: Mask the NTE when the TE AC threshold is more than 50 dB greater than the NTE BC threshold.

Many audiologists prefer to adopt one masking rule regardless of frequency, as is the case with supra-aural earphones (see below). The most defensible rule would be the most conservative IA of 50 dB:

- Mask the NTE when the TE AC threshold is more than 50 dB greater than the NTE BC threshold.

Supra-Aural Earphones

IA for supra-aural earphones is frequency-dependent and can range from 40 to 80 dB (Goldstein & Newman, 1994). Historically, audiologists have preferred one masking rule regardless of frequency. Sensibly, the rule adopted by most includes the most conservative IA of 40 dB:

- When a TE AC threshold exceeds the NTE BC threshold by 40 dB or more, mask the NTE via air conduction.

TYPE OF MASKING NOISE

Only a narrow band of noise (NBN) is necessary during pure-tone testing. This is based on the psychoacoustic concept of critical bands; energy outside the critical band will not improve the efficiency of the masker. NBN is calibrated according to the American National Standards Institute (ANSI) standards.

PROCEDURES

We chose to offer three "plateau-" masking method options. The procedures are called plateau methods because masking noise is delivered to the NTE at progressively higher intensities until a TE threshold plateau is reached. The methods are:

1. Hood plateau method (Hood, 1960)
2. Goldstein and Newman plateau method (Goldstein & Newman, 1994)
3. The Katz and Lezynski step variation of the plateau method (Katz & Lezynski, 2002)

Hood Plateau Method

1. **NTE:** Start with NBN masking at 10 dB above the NTE AC threshold.
   TE: Present the tone to the TE at threshold to re-establish threshold. If the tone is not heard, increase it in 5-dB intensity increments to establish a new TE AC threshold.
2. **NTE:** Masking increase #1; increase NTE AC masking 10 dB.
   TE: Present the tone to the TE at threshold. If the tone is not heard, increase it in 5-dB intensity increments to establish a new TE AC threshold.
3. **NTE:** Masking increase #2; increase NTE AC masking 10 dB.
   TE: Present the tone to the TE at threshold. If the tone is not heard, increase it in 5-dB intensity increments to establish a new TE AC threshold.
   - We recommend stopping when the TE AC threshold does not shift over two consecutive NTE 10-dB masking increases. This is the threshold plateau. If a plateau is never reached, a TE AC masked threshold cannot be measured. Record using the appropriate symbol (see Figure 2–1).
   - *Note.* 5 dB of shift may be due to central masking, the neural interaction of input from the TE and NTE in the brainstem. The shift from central masking is not clinically significant.

Verifying Masking Levels

You must elevate the NTE BC threshold to a level within the IA. For example, *with supra-aural ear-*

phones IA is 40 dB; we recommend adding enough masking to elevate the NTE BC threshold to within 30 dB of the TE threshold. *Note.* If the TE air conduction threshold shifts to the equipment intensity limit or patient uncomfortable level, record at that level using the appropriate no-response masking symbol (see Figure 2–1).

Goldstein and Newman Plateau Method

1. **NTE:** Start with NBN masking at 15 dB above the NTE AC threshold.
   TE: Present the tone to the TE at threshold to re-establish the TE AC threshold. If the tone is not heard, increase it in 5-dB intensity increments to establish a new TE AC threshold.
2. **NTE:** Masking increase #1; increase NTE AC masking 5 dB.
   TE: Present the tone to the TE at threshold to re-establish the TE AC threshold. If the tone is not heard, increase it in 5-dB intensity increments to establish a new TE AC threshold.
3. **NTE:** Masking increase #2; increase NTE AC masking 5 dB.
   TE: Present the tone to the TE at threshold to re-establish the TE AC threshold. If the tone is not heard, increase it in 5-dB intensity increments to establish a new TE AC threshold.
4. **NTE:** Masking increase #3; increase NTE AC masking 5 dB.
   TE: Present the tone to the TE at threshold to re-establish the TE AC threshold. If the tone is not heard, increase it in 5-dB intensity increments to establish a new TE AC threshold.
   - We recommend stopping when the TE AC threshold does not shift over

three consecutive NTE 5-dB masking increases. This is the threshold plateau. If a plateau is never reached a TE AC masked threshold cannot be measured. Record using the appropriate symbol (see Figure 2–1).

Note. Central masking can cause a 5-dB shift; this is clinically insignificant and it can be ignored.

Verifying Masking Levels

You must elevate the NTE BC threshold to a level within the IA. For example, *with supra-aural earphones*, IA is 40 dB; add enough masking to elevate the NTE BC threshold to within 30 dB of the TE threshold. *Note.* If the TE air conduction threshold shifts to the equipment intensity limit, or patient uncomfortable level, record at that level using the appropriate symbol (see Figure 2–1).

Comparison of the Hood Plateau Method and the Goldstein and Newman Plateau Method

It can be shown that 30 dB is the minimum amount of NTE AC masking you'll ever use (i.e., when there are no TE AC threshold shifts).

Hood

- 10 NTE AC masking starting level
- + 10 NTE AC masking increase #1
- + 10 NTE AC masking increase #2

= 30 dB

Goldstein and Newman

- 15 NTE AC masking starting level
- + 5 NTE AC masking increase #1
- + 5 NTE AC masking increase #2
- + 5 NTE AC masking increase #3

  = 30 dB

The Katz and Lezynski Step Variation of the Plateau Method

1. **NTE:** Start with NBN masking at 30 dB above the NTE AC threshold, the minimum amount of masking you'll ever use with the above plateau methods.
2. **TE:** Present the tone to the TE at threshold to re-establish the TE AC threshold. If the tone is heard a threshold plateau is assumed; record the TE threshold on the audiogram using the appropriate symbol (see Figure 2–1). If the tone is not heard, increase it in 5-dB increments to establish a new TE AC threshold. *Note.* Central masking can cause a 5-dB shift; this is clinically insignificant and it can be ignored.
3. **NTE:** If threshold shifts, add 20 dB more masking (the equivalent of two Hood steps) and retest the TE AC threshold. If the tone is heard, a threshold plateau is reached; record threshold using the appropriate symbol (see Figure 2–1). If the tone is not heard, increase it in 5-dB intensity increments to establish a new TE AC threshold. Additional masking will then be required. Continue in this manner until the TE AC threshold does not shift more than 5 dB with the addition of masking. If a plateau is never reached, a

TE AC masked threshold cannot be measured. Record using the appropriate symbol (see Figure 2–1).

Verifying Masking Levels

You must elevate the NTE BC threshold to a level within the IA. For example, *with supra-aural earphones* IA is 40 dB; add enough masking to elevate the NTE BC threshold to within 30 dB of the TE threshold. *Note.* If the TE air conduction threshold shifts to the equipment intensity limit, or patient uncomfortable level, record at that level using the appropriate symbol (see Figure 2–1).

OVERMASKING

Overmasking occurs when NTE *masking noise* crosses to the TE at an audible level. For example, *with supra-aural earphones*, masking noise will cross to the TE, but it will be attenuated by the IA of 40 dB. If the noise level reaches the TE at or above the TE BC threshold, it will mask the TE. By definition, this is "overmasking." In such cases, a masked TE threshold cannot be measured.

CENTRAL MASKING

As discussed above, a 5-dB TE threshold shift may be due to central masking, the neural interaction of input from the TE and NTE in the brainstem. The shift from central masking is not clinically significant.

REFERENCES

Goldstein, B., & Newman, C. (1994). Clinical masking: A decision-making process. In J. Katz (Ed.), *Handbook of clinical audiology* (4th ed., pp. 109–131). Baltimore, MD: Williams & Wilkins.

Hood, J. D. (1960). The principles and practice of bone-conduction audiometry. *Laryngoscope*, *70*, 1211–1228.

Katz, J. & Lezynski, J. (2002). Clinical masking. In J. Katz (Ed.), *Handbook of clinical audiology* (5th ed., pp. 124–141). Baltimore, MD: Lippincott Williams & Wilkins.

Yacullo, W. (2009). Clinical masking. In J. Katz, L. Medwetsky, R. Burkard, & L. Hood (Eds.), *Handbook of clinical audiology* (6th ed., pp. 80–115). Baltimore, MD: Lippincott Williams & Wilkins.

5

Pure-Tone Bone Conduction Masking

THE PROBLEM

A tone presented through a bone vibrator to the test ear (TE) mastoid can "crossover" and be heard in the non-test ear (NTE). How does it cross over? Bone-conducted (BC) sound waves of sufficient intensity vibrate the skull and skull contents including both cochlea. When you present a bone-conducted tone we assume the worst case (most conservative) scenario of 0 dB IA: a tone presented through a bone vibrator will reach each cochlea at the same intensity. Therefore, in many cases, the audiologist cannot discern whether an unmasked BC threshold reflects hearing sensitivity in the right ear, the left ear, or both.

MASKING

We deliver noise to mask one ear so we can test the other ear. For example, masking delivered 30 dB above a NTE AC threshold will elevate that ear's AC threshold *and* NTE BC threshold by 30 dB. With sufficient masking the NTE threshold will be elevated to a level rendering it unable to hear test tones.

WHEN TO MASK

Mask when there is a ≥15 "air-bone gap":

- An air-bone gap is when TE BC threshold is at least 15 dB better than the TE AC threshold *in the same ear.*
- For any ear with an air-bone gap, retest the bone-conduction threshold while masking the NTE via air conduction.

TYPE OF MASKING NOISE

Only a narrow band of noise (NBN) is necessary during pure-tone testing. This is based on the psychoacoustic concept of critical bands; energy outside the critical band will not improve efficiency of the masker. NBN is calibrated according to American National Standards Institute (ANSI) standards.

TRANSDUCERS

Typically, the bone vibrator is placed on the TE mastoid, and a supra-aural or insert earphone is used on the NTE.

PROCEDURES

We chose to offer three "plateau-" masking method options. The procedures are called plateau methods because masking noise is delivered to the NTE at progressively higher intensities until a TE threshold plateau is reached. The methods are:

1. Hood plateau method (Hood, 1960)
2. Goldstein and Newman plateau method (Goldstein & Newman, 1994)
3. The Katz and Lezynski step variation of the Hood plateau method (Katz & Lezynski, 2002)

Hood Plateau Method

1. **NTE:** Start with NBN masking at 10 dB, *plus the amount of the occlusion effect* above the NTE AC threshold. We recommend the following amounts be added for the occlusion effect:
   - When masking with insert earphones: Add 10 dB of masking when testing at 250 Hz (Yacullo, 1996).
   - When masking with supra-aural earphones: Add 30 dB of masking at 250 Hz, 20 dB of masking at 500 Hz, and 10 dB of masking at 1000 Hz (Yacullo, 1996).
   - Or instead of using average occlusion effect data, you can measure occlusion effect for each patient (Dean & Martin, 2000):
     - Place BC vibrator on the test mastoid and measure the unoccluded BC thresholds.

- ➤ Place earphone in/on NTE and re-measure BC thresholds with no masking.
- ➤ The occlusion effect is the difference between the occluded and unoccluded BC thresholds.

TE: Present the BC tone to the test mastoid (TE) at threshold to re-establish threshold. If the tone is not heard, increase it in 5-dB intensity increments to establish a new TE BC threshold.

2. **NTE:** Masking increase #1; increase NTE AC masking 10 dB.
   TE: Present the BC tone to the TE at threshold. If the tone is not heard, increase it in 5 dB increments to establish a new TE BC threshold.
3. **NTE:** Masking increase #2; increase NTE AC masking 10 dB.
   TE: Present the BC tone to the TE at threshold. If the tone is not heard, increase it in 5-dB increments to establish a new TE BC threshold.
   - We recommend stopping when the TE BC threshold does not shift over two consecutive NTE 10-dB masking increases. This is the threshold plateau. If a plateau is never reached a TE BC masked threshold cannot be measured. Record using the appropriate symbol (see Figure 2–1).
   - *Note.* A shift of 5 dB may be due to central masking, the neural interaction of input from the TE and NTE in the brainstem. The shift from central masking is not clinically significant.

Verifying Masking Levels

- You must elevate the NTE BC threshold until it cannot participate in testing. This will occur when the NTE BC threshold is elevated to at least 10 dB greater than the TE BC threshold.
- *Note.* If the TE BC threshold continues to shift until no response is obtained at equipment intensity limits, a masked threshold cannot be measured. Record at that level using the appropriate masking symbol (see Figure 2–1).

Goldstein and Newman Plateau Method

1. **NTE:** Start with NBN masking at 15 dB, *plus the amount of the occlusion effect* above the NTE AC threshold
   TE: Present the BC tone to the TE at threshold to re-establish the TE BC threshold. If the tone is not heard, increase it in 5-dB intensity increments to establish a new TE BC threshold.
2. **NTE:** Masking increase #1; increase NTE AC masking 5 dB.
   TE: Present the BC tone to the TE at threshold to re-establish the TE BC threshold. If the tone is not heard, increase it in 5-dB intensity increments to establish a new TE BC threshold.
3. **NTE:** Masking increase #2; increase NTE AC masking 5 dB.
   TE: Present the BC tone to the TE at threshold to re-establish the TE BC threshold. If the tone is not heard, increase it in 5-dB intensity increments to establish a new TE BC threshold.

4. **NTE:** Masking increase #3; increase NTE AC masking 5 dB.
   TE: Present the BC tone to the TE at threshold to re-establish the TE BC threshold. If the tone is not heard, increase it in 5-dB increments to establish a new TE BC threshold.

Verifying Masking Levels

- You must elevate the NTE BC threshold until it cannot participate in testing. This will occur when the NTE BC threshold is elevated to at least 10 dB greater than the TE BC threshold.
- *Note.* If the TE BC threshold continues to shift until no response is obtained at equipment intensity limits, a masked threshold cannot be measured. Record at that level using the appropriate masking symbol (see Figure 2–1).

Comparison of the Hood Plateau Method and the Goldstein and Newman Plateau Method

It can be shown that 30 dB is the minimum amount of NTE AC masking you'll ever use (when there are no TE AC threshold shifts).

Hood

- 10 NTE AC masking starting level
- + 10 NTE AC masking increase #1
- + 10 NTE AC masking increase #2
  = 30 dB

Goldstein and Newman

- 15 NTE AC masking starting level
- + 5 NTE AC masking increase #1
- + 5 NTE AC masking increase #2
- + 5 NTE AC masking increase #3

  = 30 dB

The Katz and Lezynski Step Variation of the Plateau Method

1. **NTE:** Start with NBN masking at 30dB, *plus the amount of the occlusion effect* above the NTE AC threshold, the minimum amount of masking you'll ever use (when there are no threshold shifts).
2. **TE:** Present the BC tone to the TE at threshold to re-establish the TE BC threshold. If the tone is heard a plateau is assumed; record the TE BC threshold on the audiogram using the appropriate symbol (see Figure 2–1). *Note.* If the tone is not heard, increase it in 5-dB increments to establish a new TE BC threshold. A shift of 5 dB may be attributable to central masking, and therefore this amount of shift may be ignored.
3. **NTE:** If threshold TE BC threshold shifts >5 dB, add 20 dB more masking (the equivalent of two Hood steps) and retest the TE BC threshold. If the tone is heard, a plateau is reached; record threshold using the appropriate symbol see (see Figure 2–1). If the tone is not heard, increase it in 5-dB increments to establish a new TE BC threshold. Continue in this manner until the TE BC threshold does not shift with added masking

(a threshold plateau is reached). Record threshold using the appropriate symbol (see Figure 2–1).

Verifying Masking Levels

- You must elevate the NTE BC threshold until it cannot participate in testing. This will occur when the NTE BC threshold is elevated to at least 10 dB greater than the TE BC threshold.
- *Note.* If the TE BC threshold continues to shift until no response is obtained at equipment intensity limits, a masked threshold cannot be measured. Record at that level using the appropriate masking symbol (see Figure 2–1).

OVERMASKING

Overmasking occurs when NTE masking noise crosses to the TE at an audible level. For example, *with supra-aural earphones,* masking noise will cross to the TE, but it will be attenuated by the IA of 40 dB. If the noise level reaches the TE at or above the TE BC threshold, it will mask the TE. By definition, this is "overmasking." In such cases, a masked TE threshold cannot be measured.

CENTRAL MASKING

As discussed above, 5 dB of shift may be due to central masking, the neural interaction of input from the

TE and NTE in the brainstem. The shift from central masking is not clinically significant.

REFERENCES

Dean, M., & Martin, F. (2000). Insert earphone depth and the occlusion effect. *American Journal of Audiology, 9*, 131–134. http://dx.doi.org/10.1044/1059-0889(2000/011)

Goldstein, B., & Newman, C. (1994). Clinical masking: A decision-making process. In J. Katz (Ed.), *Handbook of clinical audiology* (4th ed., pp. 109–131). Baltimore, MD: Williams & Wilkins.

Hood, J. D. (1960). The principles and practice of bone-conduction audiometry. *Laryngoscope, 70*, 1211–1228.

Katz, J. & Lezynski, J. (2002). Clinical masking. In J. Katz (Ed.), *Handbook of clinical audiology* (5th ed., pp. 124–141). Baltimore, MD: Lippincott Williams & Wilkins.

Yacullo, W. (1996). *Clinical masking procedures*. Needham Heights, MA: Allyn & Bacon.

6

Speech Recognition Threshold (SRT)

SRT

An SRT stands for speech recognition threshold, speech reception threshold (outdated term), or spondee recognition threshold (when spondees are used). Spondees: the typical stimuli for adults and most children. Spondees are two-syllable words with approximately equal stress on each syllable. Two syllable words have redundancy making them relatively easy to recognize. The spondees used have been shown by research to be familiar and homogenous with respect to audibility. Moreover, energy at 500 to 2000 Hz is most important for identification of spondees.

THRESHOLD DEFINED

An SRT is the minimum intensity level required for 50% recognition when spondees are used. A response mode is typically verbal, but for younger children, finger-pointing tasks may be used (see below).

SRT PURPOSE

An SRT is a reliability (agreement) check of the three-frequency pure-tone average (PTA).

SPONDEE PRESENTATION METHOD

Option 1: Recorded Speech

Advantages of recorded speech have been discussed since 1946 (Carhart). The ASHA (1988), and more recently, Roeser and Clark (2008), recommended recorded speech. The authors concur. Recorded is best practice because "the words are not the test, the recording is the test" (unknown source). Recorded spondees allow intensity, articulation, and accent to be standardized. Computer audiometers often have calibrated digital speech files. However, when using speech recorded on CDs, audiologists must calibrate by adjusting a 1000 Hz calibration tone at the beginning of the recording to 0 dB on VU the meter. All spondees will then peak at or near zero on the VU meter, meaning the spondees will be at the test intensity selected +/− 3 dB.

Option 2: Monitored Live Voice (MLV)

The most common choice is monitored live voice (Martin, Champlin, & Chambers, 1998). The term "live voice" means spondees are spoken into the audiometer microphone by the audiologist. It is "monitored" because the audiologist must peak presentation intensity to within +/− 3 dB of the target 0 dB on the VU meter. If accomplished the spondees will be at the test intensity selected +/− 3 dB, but this can be a difficult task that requires practice.

BEST PRACTICE: FAMILIARIZATION

Spondees are chosen to be familiar, but familiarity can be assured by asking patients to repeat an alphabetized spondee list heard at a comfortably loud level. The audiologist can eliminate words that the patient has difficulty with prior to testing. Tillman and Jerger (1959) found a 4- to 5-dB SRT improvement with familiarization, and we recommend it as best practice. Unfortunately, only 53% of audiologists familiarize (Martin, 1994).

SRT PROCEDURE

The routine clinical test battery includes obtaining an SRT in each ear separately under earphones. Traditionally we test the better ear first, and if no better ear is suspected, default to testing the right ear first.

SRT Procedure Instructions

Instruction for SRT measurement can be similar to those for pure-tone threshold measurement. Instruct patients on the nature of task (speech threshold test), the type of material used (two-syllable words), the mode of response (repeat the words), and respond to soft words (guess when unsure).

Martin and Dowdy SRT Procedure

Martin and Dowdy (1986) described a procedure consistent with the "10 down 5 up" procedure used for pure-tone threshold evaluation.

Martin and Dowdy Preliminary Phase

Start with a spondee at 30 dB to the better ear, or the right ear if no better ear is suspected.

If your patient responds correctly, advance to the test phase. If your patient fails to respond correctly, ascend and present a spondee at 50 dB, and then in 10-dB ascending steps until a correct response is seen or the limit of the audiometer is reached.

Martin and Dowdy Test Phase

Whenever a spondee is repeated correctly, present the next spondee "10 dB down," and whenever a spondee is incorrect, present the next spondee "5 dB up."

Threshold

Threshold can be defined as lowest intensity level at which three of six (50%) spondees were repeated correctly during ascending runs (Martin & Dowdy, 1986), although most audiologists opt instead for a two of four criterion.

ASHA SRT Procedure

Although few use it, the ASHA SRT procedure is valid and reliable to measure SRT in 2-dB steps or 5-dB steps. Below we briefly describe the 2-dB step procedure.

ASHA SRT Preliminary Phase

Present a spondee 30 to 40 dB above the estimated SRT or patient's PTA. If the patient does not respond correctly, then increase the level in 20-dB steps until a correct response is obtained. When a correct response is obtained, descend in 10-dB decrements, presenting one spondee at each 10-dB decrement level until the patient responds incorrectly. Present a second spondee at that level. Identify the level at which two consecutive spondees are missed.

ASHA 2-dB SRT Test Phase

The test phase starting level will be 10 dB above the level at which two consecutive spondees were missed. Present two spondees at the starting level and at each successive 2-dB decrement. Testing is completed when five out of the first six spondees are repeated correctly and five out of the last six spondees are repeated incorrectly. *Note.* If five out of the first six spondees are *not* repeated correctly, the starting level was insufficient; we recommend a 10-dB higher starting level. The ASHA 2-dB SRT threshold calculation is the starting level in dB minus the total number of spondees correctly repeated plus one (Table 6–1).

Table 6–1. Example of ASHA 2-dB SRT Search

Starting Phase	*First Spondee Response*	*Second Spondee Response*
50 dB	Correct response	
40 dB	Correct response	
30 dB	Correct response	
20 dB	Correct response	
10 dB	Incorrect response	Incorrect response
Testing Phase	***First Spondee Response***	***Second Spondee Response***
20 dB starting level	Correct response	Correct response
18 dB	Correct response	Correct response
16 dB	Correct response	Incorrect response
14 dB	Incorrect response	Incorrect response
12 dB	Incorrect response	Incorrect response

Threshold calculation formula: Starting level minus the total number correct + 1 = SRT

Threshold calculation in this example: 20 – 5 + 1 = 16 dB

INTERPRETATION

The audiometer is calibrated so the SRT and the PTA should be similar, that is, they should "agree." Good, fair, and poor agreements are given below:

- SRT within 0 to 6 dB of PTA = good agreement

- SRT within 7 to 12 dB of PTA = fair agreement
- SRT and PTA differing by >13 dB = poor agreement

What Does SRT-PTA Agreement Mean?

- Good SRT-PTA agreement suggests the PTA is reliable.
- Therefore, the audiogram is likely to be valid, since reliability is a requirement for validity.

What Might SRT-PTA Disagreement Mean?

Possibilities include:

- Nonorganic hearing loss
- Misunderstood instructions or biased responses
- Poor test techniques
- Poor speech understanding: neural site-of-lesion, cognitive or language disorder
- Precipitously sloping hearing loss requiring use of two-frequency PTA
- Equipment malfunction or poor earphone placement

SRT MODIFICATIONS FOR CHILDREN

The ASHA's SRT guideline (1988) includes a list of spondaic words appropriate for most children aged 5 to 12 years. These words can be represented pictorially, and if so, should be appropriate for children with a developmental age under 6 years. For some children, it may be advantageous to use items in the room, or body parts in lieu of standardized spondaic words. Example modifications for children include:

Picture Spondee Threshold Test (PSTT)

Audiologists use monitored live voice to deliver the spondees represented in the PSTT booklet viewed by the child. The patient response task is four alternative-forced choices (picture pointing task). We recommend an assistant hold the booklet, turn the pages, and report responses to the audiologist.

Informal Pointing to Body Parts

For some children it might be advantageous to use body parts known to the child. For example, the child may be asked to point to his nose, ear, hair, eyes, chin, feet, and so forth.

REFERENCES

American Speech-Language-Hearing Association. (1988). Guidelines for determining threshold level for speech. *ASHA*, *30*, 85–89.

Carhart, R. (1946). Monitored live-voice as a test of auditory acuity. *Journal of the Acoustical Society of America*, *17*, 339. http://dx.doi.org/10.1121/1.1916338

Conn, M. J., Dancer, J., & Ventry, I. M. (1975). A spondee list for determining speech reception threshold without prior familiarization. *Journal of Speech and Hearing Disorders*, *40*, 388–396.

Martin, F. N. (1994). *Introduction to audiology* (5th ed.). Boston, MA: Allyn & Bacon.

Martin, F. N., Champlin, C. A., & Chambers, J. A. (1998). Seventh survey of audiometric practices in the United States. *Journal of the American Academy of Audiology, 9,* 95–104.

Martin, F. N., & Dowdy, L. (1986). A modified spondee threshold procedure. *Journal of Auditory Research, 26,* 115–119.

Roeser, R. J., & Clark, J. L. (2008). Live voice speech recognition audiometry—stop the madness! *Audiology Today, 20,* 32–33.

Tillman, T. W., & Jerger, J. F. (1959). Some factors affecting the spondee threshold in normal-hearing subjects. *Journal of Speech, Language, and Hearing Research, 2,* 141–146.

7

Speech Recognition Threshold Masking

THE PROBLEM

Speech presented through an earphone to the test ear (TE) can cross over and be heard in the non-test ear (NTE). Air conducted (AC) sound waves of sufficient intensity vibrate the cartilaginous and bony external auditory meatus of the test ear, and sound waves travel by bone conduction (BC) to both the test ear and non-test ear cochlea.

MASKING

We deliver noise through an earphone to the NTE to "mask" it, that is, to elevate the NTE threshold so that the patient will not be able to hear or understand words that have crossed over. For example, masking delivered 30 dB above the NTE AC threshold will elevate the NTE AC threshold *and* NTE BC threshold by 30 dB. With sufficient masking, the

NTE threshold will be elevated to a level rendering it unable to hear test stimuli.

WHEN TO MASK

When sound crosses from the TE to the NTE, it will be attenuated by the skull and skull contents. The amount of attenuation, called interaural attenuation (IA), is 60 dB for insert earphones, 45 dB for supra-aural earphones (Yacullo, 2009).

Insert Earphones

Mask the NTE when the TE AC unmasked SRT is more than 60 dB greater than the best NTE BC pure-tone threshold between 500 to 4000 Hz. The best NTE BC pure-tone threshold is limited to 500 to 4000 Hz because those frequencies are most important for understanding speech.

Supra-Aural Earphones

Mask the NTE when the TE AC unmasked SRT is more than 45 dB greater than the best NTE BC pure-tone threshold between 500 to 4000 Hz.

TYPE OF MASKING NOISE

Speech noise is a calibrated broadband spectrum of noise concentrated in the 300 to 3000 Hz range.

MASKING STARTING LEVEL

Masking Level for Insert Earphones (Martin & Clark, 2015)

TE unmasked SRT

– 50 dB*

+ the largest NTE air-bone gap

= Starting masking level presented to NTE

*Reduces the difference between the ears to less than the 60 dB IA

Masking Level for Supra-Aural Earphones (Martin & Clark, 2015)

TE unmasked SRT

– 35 dB*

+ the largest NTE air-bone gap

= Starting masking level presented to NTE

*Reduces the difference between the ears to less than the 45 dB IA

MASKING PROCEDURE

- Deliver the starting masking level to the NTE.
- Re-measure the SRT in the TE, if it does not change, stop and record.

- If SRT shifts, *add the amount of the shift* to the NTE masking and *re-measure SRT in the TE.*
- Continue in the manner until the SRT does not shift.

OVERMASKING

Overmasking occurs when NTE masking *noise* crosses to the TE at an audible level. For example, with supra-aural earphones, masking noise will cross to the TE, but it will be attenuated by the IA of 45 dB. If the noise level reaches the TE at or above the TE BC threshold, it will mask the TE. By definition, this is "overmasking." In such cases, a masked TE SRT cannot be measured.

REFERENCES

Martin, F. N., & Clark, J. G. (2015). Nonorganic hearing loss. In J. Katz (Ed.), *Handbook of clinical audiology* (7th ed., pp. 617–630). Philadelphia, PA: Wolters Kluwer.

Yacullo, W. (2009). Clinical masking. In J. Katz, L. Medwetsky, R. Burkard, & L. Hood (Eds.), *Handbook of clinical audiology* (6th ed., pp. 80–115). New York, NY: Lippincott Williams & Wilkins.

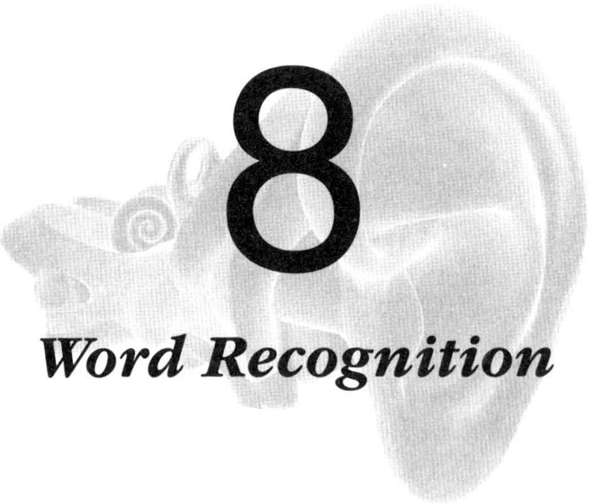

8 Word Recognition

WORD RECOGNITION

There are many supra-threshold speech tests. The most common is word recognition. The results obtained are usually called the word recognition score (WRS) and are given in percentage correct. An outdated term is word discrimination, or "discrim." A WRS is obtained using monosyllabic words presented at an audible level. The goal for diagnostic testing is to find the patient's best WRS.

WRS DIAGNOSIS AND PROGNOSIS

Diagnosis

The general testing outcomes are that patients with normal hearing do best, and patients with conductive hearing loss often do similarly well. Patients with outer hair cell disorder might do somewhat more poorly than those with normal hearing or conductive hearing loss. Finally, patients with inner hair cell and/or neural disorder almost always do most poorly.

Prognosis

The results might also help to suggest a prognosis for audiologic management and treatment. A general tendency is that the poorer the WRS, the poorer the prognosis for hearing aid use.

COMMON-WORD LIST OPTIONS

The criteria for word selection and list construction are beyond the scope and purpose of this text. Suffice it to say that phonetic or phonemic balancing, homogeneity among words, and homogeneity among word lists, were important considerations when word lists were created. The two most commonly used include the Northwestern University #6 (Tillman and Carhart, 1966) word lists (four 50-word lists), and the somewhat easier Central Institute for the Deaf (CID) W-22 word lists (Hirsh, Davis, Silverman, Reynolds, and Benson, 1952) (four 50-word lists).

Note. A carrier phrase is included prior to each word to prepare the patient. Common-carrier phrases include "say the word" and "you will say."

FULL- LIST OR HALF-LIST PRESENTATION

The original researchers of the NU#6 and W-22 word lists intended a full 50-word list to be given to each ear. However, many audiologists believe 25 word half- lists to each ear are more efficient and provide acceptable results.

Supporting Full-List Presentation

The NU#6 and W-22 word lists are phonetically or phonemically balanced, depending on the word lists. Phonetic or phonemic balance is maintained only with a full 50-word list. Moreover, test–retest reliability is minimally better with full 50-word lists (Thornton & Raffin, 1978).

Supporting Half-List Presentation

Most audiologists do half-lists (Martin, Champlin, & Chamgers, 1998). Although phonetic or phonemic balancing requires full lists, it does not affect WRS (Martin, Champlin, & Perez, 2000; Tobias, 1964), and half-lists are reliable (Thornton & Raffin, 1978). We recommend 25-word lists. An alternative approach was recommended by Runge and Hosford-Dunn (1985):

- If after 10 words, the WRS is 100%, stop and record 10 word WRS.
- If after 25 words, the WRS is at least 84%, stop and record 25 word WRS.
- If after 25 words, the WRS is less than 84%, finish and record the 50 word WRS.

PRESENTATION MODE: LIVE VOICE OR RECORDED WORDS

The most common choice is monitored live voice (MLV). The rationale often given for MLV is that it is fast, easy, and usually accurate. However, recorded presentation is better, and this has been reported since 1946 (Carhart) and as recently as 2008 (Roeser & Clark, 2008). Recorded words afford standardized word intensity, articulation, and accent.

PROCEDURES

Instructions: ASHA guidelines

Instruct patients on the nature of the task (word recognition test), type of material used (one-syllable words), mode of response (repeat the words), and to respond to soft words (guess).

Familiarization

Unlike SRT testing, do not familiarize for WRS.

WRS Presentation Level

The goal is usually to present words at a level that will yield patients' maximum WRS, called "PB max" (Phonetic/phonemic Balance Maximum WRS). The problem is that there is no single presentation level *guaranteed* to yield PB Max. Therefore, we must choose an initial presentation level.

- Research has shown that 30 to 40 dBSL (30 to 40 dB above the SRT or above the PTA) is likely to yield PB Max for most normally hearing listeners, so 30 dB SL, 35 dB SL, or 40 dB SL would all be reasonable initial presentation levels. Dennis, Beck, Chandler, and Schafer (2004) recommended 40 dB, but adding more as needed to ensure presentation level is at least 5 dB greater than the air conduction pure-tone threshold at 2000 Hz.

- Martin and Clark (2015) offered the patient's most comfortable listening level (MCL) +5 to 10 dB.
- Guthrie and Mackersie (2009) suggested the loudness discomfort level (LDL) −5 dB.

Proponents of these and other presentation levels provide their rationales, and the interested reader should explore them in the literature. Any reasonable level can be used initially; what is most important is that if one suspects PB max has not been measured, further testing should be considered.

Determining If PB Max Has Been Measured

We offer three ways to determine whether PB max (or close to it) has been measured.

1. If WRS is at least 84%, assume you have found PB max or close to it (Runge & Hosford-Dunn, 1985). We recommend this.
2. Another tool is the data from Dubno, Lee, Klein, Matthews, and Lam (1995), which shows the lowest acceptable (95% confidence limit) WRS for a given three-frequency PTA (Table 8–1).
3. Finally, Dennis, Beck, Chandler, and Schafer (2004) and The Department of Veterans Affairs (2011) recommended presenting a 25-word list 6 dB above the initial presentation level, and a 25-word list 6 dB below the initial presentation

Table 8–1. The Lowest Acceptable (95% Confidence Limit) Word Recognition Score (WRS) for Given Three-Frequency Pure-Tone Average (PTA) at 500 Hz, 1000 Hz, and 2000 Hz (Dubno, Lee, Klein, Matthews, & Lam, 1995)

Three-Frequency PTA	*Lowest Acceptable WRS in Percentage*
0	100
4	96
8	96
12	92
16	88
20	88
24	84
28	76
32	72
36	68
40	64
44	56
48	52
52	48
56	44
60	36
64	32
68	24
72	24
76	12
80	12
84	8
88 or poorer	0

level. If WRS does not change more than 4%, stop and assume you have found PB max (or close to it). Record the highest WRS.

Searching for PB Max

As stated, we recommend a PB max search when WRS is less than 84%. To conduct a PB max search, increase (or decrease) test intensity 10 dB and retest WRS. Stop when WRS stabilizes +/− 4% or when it meets or exceeds 84%. Throughout this process, audiologists must take care not to exceed patients' LDL.

WRS INTERPRETATION

Once PB max has been established, the percentage correct score can be categorized with descriptors. The following descriptors by Goetzinger (1978) are an option:

- 90% to100% = Normal limits
- 75% to 90% = Slight difficulty
- 60% to 75% = Moderate difficulty
- 50% to 60% = Poor recognition
- <50% = Very poor recognition

WRS and PTA

WRS scores that are poorer than expected for the audiogram might be considered a red flag for VIII nerve or more central disorders. The Dubno, Lee, Klein, Matthews, and Lam's (1995) 95% confidence limits given in Table 8–1 can be a useful tool for determining if WRS is poorer than expected for the PTA.

WRS and Asymmetry

Asymmetry is another diagnostic red flag. Thornton and Raffin's (1978) 95% confidence limits (Table 8–2) can be a useful tool for ear-to-ear comparisons, and it can also be used to assess year-to-year changes. For more on the topic of asymmetry, see the medical referral in Chapter 27.

CLINICAL DECISION MAKING

Resist the temptation to be too rigid in your use of norms, including the Dubno, Lee, Klein, Matthews, and Lam (1995) data, and the Thornton and Raffin's (1978) data. Norms are tools used by clinicians, but remember that clinicians make decision and tools do not.

WRS MIGHT BE A WEAK DIAGNOSTIC TEST

Wiley, Stoppenbach, Feldhake, Moss, and Thordardottir (1995) provides the interested reader with an overview of potential weaknesses of using WRS diagnostically. Suffice it to say other tests might provide better diagnostic sensitivity and specificity for identifying sensory and neural disorder. However, tradition and reimbursement issues will likely dictate the continued measurement of WRS for the foreseeable future.

Table 8–2. Acceptable Word Recognitions Score (WRS) Asymmetry or Test–Retest Difference (Thornton & Raffin, 1978)

Word Recognition Score in Percentages	***When Using 50–Word Lists***	***When Using 25–Word Lists***
100	96–100	92–100
98	90–100	
96	86–100	80–100
94	82–98	
92	78–98	72–100
90	76–98	
88	74–96	68–96
86	70–96	
84	68–94	60–96
82	66–94	
80	64–92	56–96
78	60–92	
76	58–90	52–92
74	56–88	
72	54–86	48–92
70	52–86	
68	50–84	44–88
66	48–82	
64	46–80	40–84
62	44–78	
60	42–78	36–84
58	40–76	
56	38–74	32–80
54	36–72	
52	34–70	28–76

continues

Table 8–2. *continued*

Word Recognition Score in Percentages	*When Using 50–Word Lists*	*When Using 25–Word Lists*
50	32–68	
48	30–66	24–72
46	28–64	
44	26–62	20–68
42	24–60	
40	22–58	16–64
38	22–56	
36	20–54	16–60
34	18–52	
32	16–50	12–56
30	14–48	
28	14–46	8–52
26	12–44	
24	10–42	8–48
22	8–40	
20	8–36	4–44
18	6–34	
16	6–32	4–40
14	4–30	
12	4–26	4–32
10	2–24	
8	2–22	0–28
6	2–18	
4	0–14	0–20
2	0–10	
0	0–4	0–8

PHONEMIC SCORING

Phonemic scoring involves identifying the specific phonemes patients miss during testing. Phonemic scoring has lost favor in current practice, but it was once used in counseling/treatment, for example to suggest lip-reading goals. Other word lists better suited to this are available, but beyond the scope of this text.

ROLLOVER

Patients with VIII or low brainstem lesions almost always do relatively poorly on word recognition tests. They might do even worse when their neurons are stressed with high intensity presentation levels. When a patient does significantly worse at higher intensities, the WRS is said to have "rolled over."

When Should You Test Rollover?

This clinical decision can be complicated, but it can be condensed into this simple rule: Consider testing for rollover when the audiogram suggests sensory/neural hearing loss, and you want to assess the extent to which there is neural involvement.

Rollover Procedure Options

We propose two options:

- Option 1: Present a word list (typically 25 words) at LDL −5 dB.

- Option 2: Present a word list (typically 25 words) at 90 dB HL if tolerable (Martin & Clark, 2015).

As with the initial starting level, clinical judgment is involved in choosing a level for testing rollover. The intensity level must be greater than the level at which PB max was obtained, but it must not exceed patients' LDLs.

The "Rollover Index" (RI) Calculation

- (PB maximum − PB minimum) ÷ PB maximum

For example, suppose a patient's PB max was 76%, and he or she scored 36% when the intensity level was increased:

- (76% − 36%) ÷ 76%
- RI = 0.53

A RI of 0.53 is significant, raising suspicion of VIII nerve or brainstem disorder (see RI norms below).

Another example: Suppose a patient's PB max was 64%, and he or she scored 50% when the intensity level was increased.

- (64% − 50%) ÷ 64%
- RI = 0.22

A RI of 0.22 is *not* significant (see RI norms and interpretation below). One could consider testing at even higher levels (if possible) to search for rollover, but

0.22 is so far from significant that the astute clinician would likely stop testing.

RI Norms

- Jerger and Jerger (1971) recommended RI ≥0.45 as significant for neural involvement.
- Silman and Silverman (1991) recommendations were RI ≥0.35 for NU#6 words and RI ≥0.35 for the somewhat easier W-22 words.

REFERENCES

American Speech-Language-Hearing Association. (1988). Guidelines for determining threshold level for speech. *ASHA*, *30*, 85–89.

Carhart, R. (1946). Monitored live-voice as a test of auditory acuity. *The Journal of the Acoustical Society of America*, *17*, 339. http://dx.doi.org/10.1121/1.1916338

Dennis, K. C., Beck, L. B., Chandler, D. W., & Schafer, J. (2004). *VHA audiology handbook, 2004, C&P exams, word recognition*. Retrieved from https://veteranclaims.wordpress.com/2011/09/01/va-audiology-handbook-2004-cp-exams-word-recognition/

Department of Veterans Affairs. (2011). *VHA audiology and speech-language pathology services*. Retrieved from https://www.google.com/?gws_rd=ssl#q=http:%2F%2Fwww.va.gov%2Fvhapublications%2FViewPublication.asp%3Fpub_ID%3D2397

Dubno, J. R., Lee, F., Klein, A., Matthews, L., & Lam, C. F. (1995). Confidence limits for maximum word-recognition scores. *Journal of Speech and Hearing Research*, *38*, 490–502.

Goetzinger. C. (1978). Word discrimination testing. In J. Katz, (Ed.), *Handbook of clinical audiology* (2nd ed., p. 155). Baltimore, MD: Williams & Wilkins.

Guthrie, L. A., & Mackersie, C. L. (2009). A comparison of presentation levels to maximize word recognition scores. *Journal of the American Academy of Audiology 20*(6), 381–390.

Hirsh, I. J., Davis, H., Silverman, S. R., Reynolds, E. G., Eldert, E., & Benson, R. W., (1952). Development of materials for speech audiometry. *Journal of Speech and Hearing Disorders, 17*, 321–337.

Jerger, J., & Jerger, S. (1971). Diagnostic significance of PB word functions. *Archives of Otolaryngology, 93*, 573–580.

Martin, F. N., Champlin, C. A., & Chambers, J. A. (1998). Seventh survey of audiometric practices in the United States. *Journal of the American Academy of Audiology, 9*, 95–104.

Martin, F. N., Champlin, C. A., & Perez, D. D. (2000). The question of phonetic balance in word recognition testing. *Journal of the American Academy of Audiology, 11*, 489–493.

Martin, F. N., & Clark, J. G. (2015). *Introduction to audiology* (12th ed.) Boston, MA: Pearson.

Roeser, R. J., & Clark, J. L. (2008). Live voice speech recognition audiometry-stop the madness! *Audiology Today. 20*, 32–33.

Runge, C. A., & Hosford-Dunn, H. (1985). Word recognition performance with modified CID W-22 word lists. *Journal of Speech, Language, and Hearing Research, 28*, 355–362. http://dx.doi.org/10.1044/jshr.2803.355

Thornton, A. R., & Raffin, M. J. M. (1978). Speech-discrimination scores modeled as a binomial variable. *Journal of Speech, Language, and Hearing Research, 21*, 507–518. http://dx.doi.org/10.1044/jshr.2103.507

Tillman, T. W., & Carhart, R. (1966). An expanded test for speech discrimination utilizing CNC monosyllabic words: Northwestern University auditory test no. 6. Technical report no. SAM-TR-66-55. San Antonio, TX,

USAF School of Aerospace Medicine, Brooks Air Force Base.

Tobias, J. V. (1964). On phonemic analysis of speech discrimination tests. *Journal of Speech and Hearing Research*, 7, 90–100.

Silman, S., & Silverman, C. (1991). *Auditory diagnosis: Principles and applications*. San Diego, CA: Academic Press.

Wiley, T. L., Stoppenbach, D. T., Feldhake, L. J., Moss, K. A., & Thordardottir, E. T. (1994). Audiologic practices: What is popular versus what is supported by evidence. *American Journal of Audiology*, *4*(1), 26–34.

9

Word Recognition Masking

THE PROBLEM

Speech presented through an earphone to the test ear (TE) can "cross over" and be heard in the non-test ear (NTE). Air-conducted (AC) sound waves of sufficient intensity vibrate the cartilaginous and bony external auditory meatus of the test ear, and sound waves travel by bone conduction (BC) to both the test ear and non-test ear cochlea.

MASKING

We deliver noise through an earphone to the NTE to "mask" it, that is, to elevate the NTE threshold so that the patient will not be able to hear or understand words that have crossed over. For example, masking delivered 30 dB above the NTE AC threshold will elevate the NTE AC threshold *and* NTE BC threshold by 30 dB. With sufficient masking, the

NTE threshold will be elevated to a level rendering it unable to hear test stimuli.

WHEN TO MASK

When sound crosses from the TE to the NTE, it will be attenuated by the skull and skull contents. The amount of attenuation, called interaural attenuation (IA), is 60 dB for insert earphones, 45 dB for supra-aural earphones (Yacullo, 2009).

Insert Earphones

Mask the NTE when the TE AC word presentation level is more than 60 dB greater than the best NTE BC pure-tone threshold between 500 to 4000 Hz.

Supra-Aural Earphones

Mask the NTE when the TE AC word presentation level is more than 45 dB greater than the best NTE BC pure-tone threshold between 500 to 4000 Hz. *Note.* The best NTE BC pure-tone threshold is limited to 500 to 4000 Hz because those frequencies are most important for understanding speech.

TYPE OF MASKING NOISE

Speech noise is a calibrated broadband spectrum of noise concentrated in the 300 to 3000 Hz range.

MASKING STARTING LEVEL

Masking Level for *Insert Earphones* (Martin, 1994)

TE word presentation level
– 50 dB*
+ the largest NTE air-bone gap
= Masking level

*Reduces the difference between the ears to less than the 60 dB IA

Masking Level for *Supra-Aural Earphones* (Martin, 1994)

TE word presentation level
– 35 dB*
+ the largest NTE air-bone gap
= Masking level

*Reduces the difference between the ears to less than the 45 dB IA

PROCEDURE

Deliver the masking to the NTE, and test WRS in the TE.

OVERMASKING

Overmasking occurs when NTE masking noise crosses to the TE at an audible level. For example, with supra-aural earphones, masking noise will cross to the TE, but it will be attenuated by the IA of 45 dB. If the noise level reaches the TE at or above the TE BC threshold, it will mask the TE. By definition, this is "overmasking." In such cases, a masked TE WRS cannot be measured.

REFERENCES

Martin, F. N. (1994). *Introduction to audiology* (5th ed.). Boston, MA: Allyn & Bacon.

Yacullo, W. (2009). Clinical masking. In J. Katz, L. Medwetsky, R. Burkard, & L. Hood (Eds.), *Handbook of clinical audiology* (6th ed., pp. 80–115). New York, NY: Lippincott Williams & Wilkins.

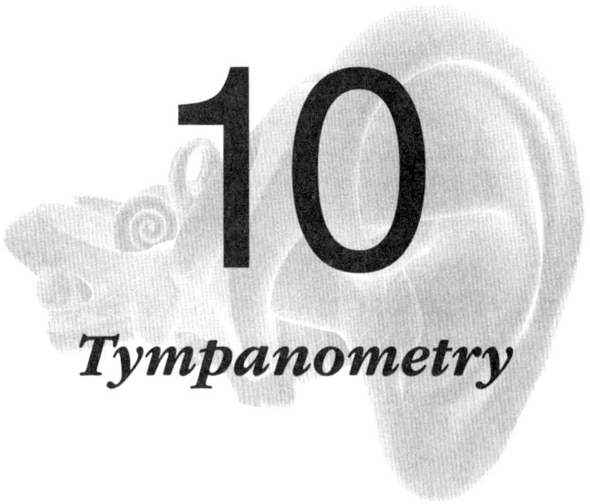

10

Tympanometry

Y226 TYMPANOMETRY

Y226 Hz tympanometry allows us to objectively evaluate the outer and middle ear. During routine tympanometry, we measure the admittance (Y) of a 226 Hz (or 220 Hz) tone through the outer and middle ear. Admittance is the ease of flow of energy, the reciprocal of impedance. Admittance is proportional to the voltage needed to maintain the 226 Hz tone in the ear canal at 85 dB SPL.

OVERVIEW, FOUR Y226 TYMPANOGRAM SUBTESTS

1. Physical volume: an indirect measure of size of the ear canal (if the tympanic membrane TM is intact) or ear canal plus middle ear (when there is a TM perforation or patent PE tube)
2. Static admittance: an indirect measure of peak TM mobility
3. Pressure peak: an indirect measure of Eustachian tube function

4. Width: an indirect measure of TM mobility but across the pressure sweep not just peak TM mobility

Subtest 1: Physical Volume AKA ECV (ear canal volume) or Vec (volume of ear canal)

Our equipment will estimate the size of the ear canal if the TM is intact. But when there is a TM perforation or patent PE tube, the measure is of the ear canal, middle ear, possibly mastoid air cells, and more if the Eustachian tube opens. The larger the physical volume, the more voltage it takes to maintain the tone at 85 dB SPL. The procedure is conducted automatically when one "runs" a tympanogram.

The Physical Volume Procedure

- Air pump: +200 daPa pressure to push the TM tight and effectively wall off the ear canal, unless there is a TM perforation or patent PE tube
- Probe speaker: 226 Hz tone
- Microphone and analysis system: The larger the canal, the more voltage it takes to maintain the tone at 85 dB SPL, and if there is a TM perforation or patent PE tube, it will take even more voltage to maintain the 85 dB SPL tone as it spreads to the middle ear and perhaps beyond. However, the data are not given in voltage. Instead, the machine estimates the physical volume in milliliters (ml), cubic centimeters (cc or cm^3) or millimhos (mmho); the three are equivalent for low-frequency tympanometry.

Normal Physical Volume

ASHA (1988) norms for adults 19 to 61 years old: 0.8 to 1.6 cm^3

ASHA (1990) norms for children 1 to 7 years: 0.3 to 0.9 cm^3

Example Ramifications. Cerumen occlusion manifesting smaller than normal ear canal might yield physical volume <0.8 cm^3 in adults and <0.3 cm^3 in in children.

Tympanic membrane perforation or patent PE tubes manifesting as a larger measurement cavity (ear canal plus middle ear space) could yield physical volumes >1.6 cm^3 in adults and >0.9 cm^3 in children.

Subtest 2: Static Admittance, AKA Peak Compensated Static Acoustic Admittance, Peak Admittance, or Static Compliance

Our equipment sweeps pressure in the ear canal from +200 to −400 daPa, all the while searching to identify maximum admittance, when the most voltage is needed to maintain the tone at 85 dB SPL. If the tympanic membrane is intact, static admittance will occur when the pressure moves the tympanic membrane into its normal and most effective position.

Static Admittance Procedure

- Air pump: sweep +200 daPa to −400 daPa
- Probe speaker: Deliver 226 Hz tone
- Microphone and analysis system: Identification of static admittance as described above. The data are provided

in an equivalent physical volume as described above, that is, in milliliters (ml), cubic centimeters (cc or cm^3) or millimhos (mmho).

Normal Static Admittance

ASHA (1988) norms for adults 19 to 61 years old: 0.3 cm^3 to 1.4 cm^3

ASHA (1990) norms for children 1 year to school age: <0.3 mmho

Example Ramifications. Middle ear effusion (otitis media) might inhibit admittance, yielding static admittance of <0.3 cm^3 in adults and children. This has been called a type B tympanogram (Figure 10–1).

Ossicular disarticulation, or a weakened tympanic membrane (monomeric/dimeric tympanic membrane), might more readily admit sound and yield static admittance of >1.4 cm^3 in adults with similar results in children. This has been called a type Ad tympanogram (see Figure 10–1).

Subtest 3: Pressure Peak

During static admittance testing described in subtest 2, the pressure at which static admittance occurs is identified in daPa. This will occur at the moment the pressure sweep moves the tympanic membrane into its normal and most effective position, more specifically when the induced ear canal pressure equals middle ear pressure. We can thus indirectly deduce middle ear pressure.

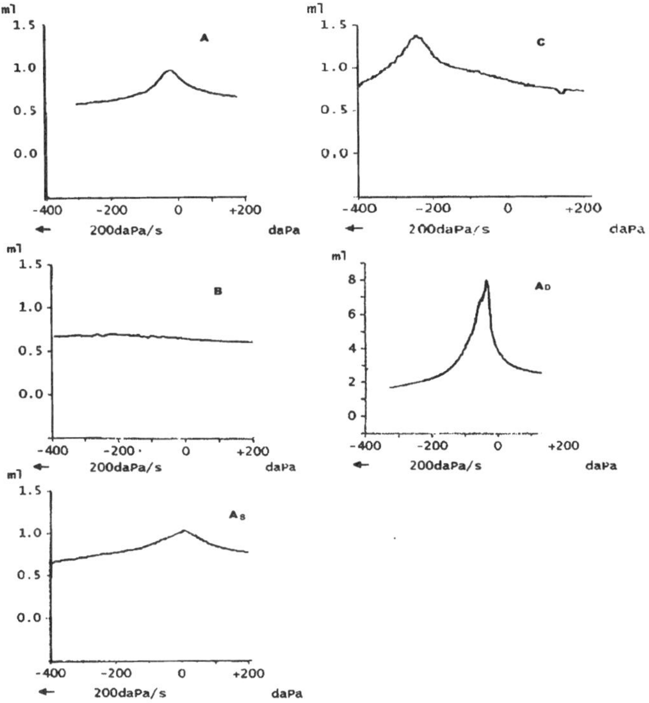

Figure 10–1. Five classic tympanogram types. From *Acoustic immittance measures* (Page 44, Figure 4–5) by L. Hunter & N. Shahnaz, 2014, San Diego, CA: Plural Publishing, Inc.

Pressure Peak Procedure

- Air pump: sweep +200 daPa to −400 daPa
- Probe speaker: delivers 226 Hz tone
- Microphone and analysis system: determines the pressure in daPa at which static admittance occurred

Normal Pressure Peak

−100 to +50 daPa. (British Society of Audiology, 2013)

Example Ramification. Eustachian tube dysfunction might yield pressure peaks of −100 daPa or poorer indicative of an improperly aerated middle ear space in adults or children. This has been called a type C tympanogram (see Figure 10–1).

Subtest 4: Width (AKA Tympanogram Width or TW)

Width is a way to quantify the shape of the tympanogram trace. Our equipment measures static admittance and pressure peak as described above, then calculates tracing width in daPa on the horizontal axis. The left-most and right-most limits of the width can be visualized as where an imaginary horizontal line intersects the tympanogram trace if the imaginary line is drawn halfway down from the peak (Figure 10–2).

Width Procedure

- Air pump: sweep +200 daPa to −400 daPa
- Probe speaker: delivers 226 Hz tone
- Microphone and analysis system: The width is identified in daPa as described above.

Normal Width

ASHA (1988) norms for adults 19 to 61 years old: 48–110 daPa

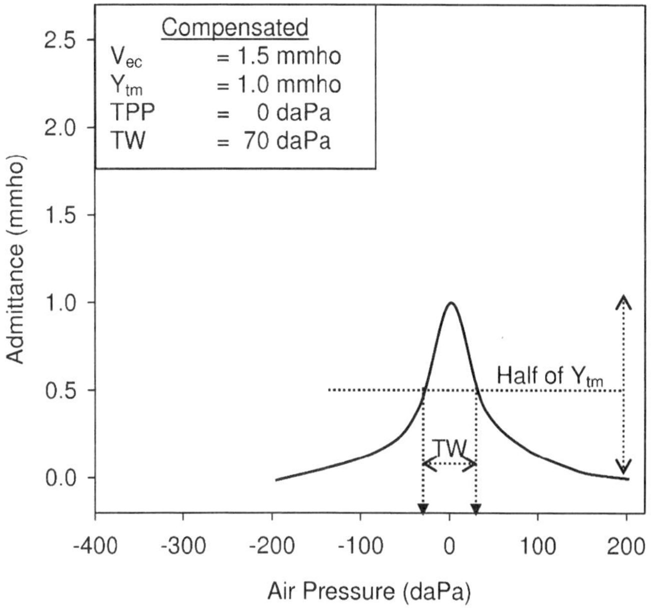

Figure 10–2. Example of a tympanogram width measure. TW is tympanogram width and Ytm is static admittance. *Audiology: Science to practice* (2nd ed.), (Page 232, Figure 8–8), by S. Kramer, 2014, San Diego, CA: Plural Publishing, Inc. Reprinted with permission.

ASHA (1990) norms for children 1 year to school age: <200 daPa.

Example Ramifications. Ossicular discontinuity and monomer/dimer typically manifest as high static admittance and widths <48 daPa.

Middle ear effusion might manifest as reduced static admittance and yield widths >110 daPa in adults and >200 daPa in children (Figure 10–3).

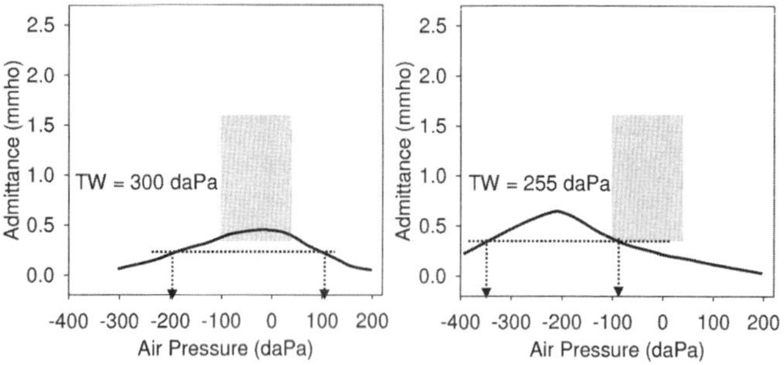

Figure 10–3. Two examples of wide tympanogram widths. From *Audiology: Science to practice* (2nd ed.), (Page 232, Figure 8–9), by S. Kramer, 2014, San Diego, CA: Plural Publishing, Inc. Reprinted with permission.

EXAMPLE TYMPANOGRAMS CASES

Normal

- History: negative
- Otoscopy: no sign of active disorder
- Audiogram: no air-bone gaps.
- Tympanogram (type A, Figure 10–1)
  - Normal physical volume
  - Normal static admittance
  - Normal pressure peak
  - Normal width

Eustachian Tube Dysfunction (ETD)

- History: possible “stuffiness”, possible upper respiratory infection (URI)
- Otoscopy: TM retraction
- Audiogram: possible small air-bone gaps; AC loss likely <7 dB (Feeney, Sanford, & Putterman, 2014), and more likely at

frequencies < 2000 Hz (Arnold & Schindler, 1963).

- Tympanogram (type C, Figure 10–1)
  - Normal physical volume
  - Normal static admittance
  - Negative pressure peak
  - Normal width

ETD with Minimal Middle Ear Effusion

- History: "stuffiness," possible URI
- Otoscopy: TM retraction, possible amber fluid or bubbles.
- Audiogram: variable, possible small air-bone gaps 5–15 dB.
- Tympanogram (type C, Figure 10–1; possible wide width)
  - Normal physical volume
  - Normal (borderline) static admittance
  - Negative pressure peak
  - Width: borderline wide

ETD with More Significant Middle Ear Effusion

- History: "stuffiness" and hearing loss, a possible URI
- Otoscopy: TM retraction and/or evidence of effusion, possible erythema
- Audiogram: air-bone gaps >15 dB
- Tympanogram (type B/wide width, Figures 10–1 and 10–3)
  - Near normal physical volume
  - Borderline normal static admittance
  - Negative pressure peak
  - Width: abnormally wide

Progressing ETD with Effusion-Filled Middle Ear Space

- History: stuffy, possible otalgia, hearing loss, possible URI
- Otoscopy: evidence of effusion, possible erythema
- Audiogram air-bone gaps up to the maximum conductive component of 60 dB
- Tympanogram (type B, Figure 10–1)
  - Normal physical volume
  - Low static admittance
  - No or minimal pressure peak (flat)
  - Flat (by definition, abnormally wide)

Effusion or Chronic Otitis Media in the Absence of Current ETD

- History: otitis media
- Otoscopy: fluid, infection, TM scarring
- Audiogram: variable air-bone gaps depending on current state of disease and middle ear damage
- Tympanogram (type B, Figure 10–1)
  - Normal physical volume
  - Low static admittance
  - Normal pressure peak
  - Width: wide

Bulging TM from Acute Otitis Media

- History: sudden otalgia, possible otorrhea and URI
- Otoscopy: bulging TM with erythema
- Audiogram: air-bone gaps

- Tympanogram
  - Normal physical volume
  - Low static admittance
  - Positive pressure peak
  - Width: likely wide

TM Perforation or Patent PE Tube

- History:
  - Perforations: head or ear trauma, chronic or acute otitis media
  - PE tubes: otitis media and ENT treatment
- Otoscopy: perforation or PE tubes
- Audiogram: variable from no air-bone gap to maximum air-bone gap depending on size and location of perforation and patency of tubes/status of otitis media
- Tympanogram
  - Large physical volume
  - Low static admittance (no peak)
  - No pressure peak
  - Flat (abnormally wide)

Complete Cerumen Occlusion

- History: stuffy with hearing loss
- Otoscopy: cerumen
- Audiogram: air-bone gaps hypothetically up to maximum of 60 dB (30–40 dB more likely)
- Tympanogram
  - Small physical volume
  - Low static admittance (no peak)
  - No pressure peak
  - Flat (abnormally wide)

Tympanic Membrane Abnormality: Monomer/Dimer, Scarring

- History: otitis media, perforation or PE tubes in the past, or trauma
- Otoscopy: monomer/dimer often appears as a darker portion of the TM with an otoscope light reflection within it. Scarring (tympanosclerosis or scar plaques) shows as white patches.
- Audiogram: normal to air-bone gaps <15 dB
- Tympanograms (type Ad, Figure 10–1)
  - Normal physical volume
  - Tympanic membrane hyperflaccidity yields high static admittance
  - Normal pressure peak
  - Normal or narrow width

Ossicular Disarticulation

- History: head or ear trauma, chronic otitis media, surgical ear
- Otoscopy: often normal, possible blood behind TM with trauma (hemotympanum)
- Audiogram: air-bone gap up to 60 dB
- Tympanogram (type Ad, Figure 10–1)
  - Normal physical volume
  - Disarticulated ossicular chain yields hyperflaccidity and high static admittance
  - Normal pressure peak
  - Normal or narrow width

Otosclerosis

- History: possible family history, female adult, gradual loss, child bearing years
- Otoscopy: normal, possible Schwartz sign (pinkish hue of the promontory)
- Audiogram: air-bone gaps with Carhart notch
- Tympanogram (narrow width)
    - Normal physical volume
    - Normal static admittance, possibly borderline low
    - Normal pressure peak
    - Width: borderline narrow or narrow

CAVEATS

One caveat of tympanometry is that different disorders might manifest with similar immittance results. For example, both otitis media and cholesteatoma could yield flat tympanograms with normal ear canal volumes. A second caveat is that lateral pathologies obscure medial pathologies. For example, a TM perforation will yield a flat tympanogram with a high ear canal volume whether or not there is otosclerosis at the stapes.

REFERENCES

American Academy of Audiology. (1997). *Identification of hearing loss & middle-ear dysfunction in preschool & school-age children.* Retrieved from http://www.audiology.org/resources/documentlibrary/Pages/HearingLossChildren.aspx

American Speech-Language-Hearing Association. (1987). *Tympanometry ASHA working group on aural acoustic-immittance measurements, committee on audiologic evaluation.* Retrieved from http://www.asha.org/policy/RP1988-00027.htm#sec1.2.4

American Speech-Language-Hearing Association. (1990). Guidelines for screening for hearing impairment and middle-ear disorders. Working group on acoustic immittance measurements and the committee on audiologic evaluation. *ASHA*, (Suppl. 2), 17–24.

Arnold, G. E., & Schindler, P., (1963). Gellé Test with Békésy audiometry: II. Normal values. *Acta Oto-Laryngologica*, *56*, 523–536. http://dx.doi.org/10.3109/00016486309127447

British Society of Audiology (2013). *Recommended procedure: Tympanometry.* Retrieved from http://www.thebsa.org.uk/wp-content/uploads/2014/04/BSA_RP_Tymp_Final_21Aug13_Final.pdf

Feeney, M. P., Sanford, C. A., & Putterman, D. B., (2014) Effects of ear-canal static pressure on pure-tone thresholds and wideband acoustic immittance. *Journal of the American Academy of Audiology*, *25*(5), 462–470.

11

Multi-Frequency and Multi-Component Tympanometry

INTRODUCTION

Middle ear admittance can be measured at multiple frequencies, and has typically been measured at 226 Hz, 678 Hz, and 1000 Hz. Tympanometry using 226 Hz probe tones was discussed in Chapter 10; in this chapter we will focus on tympanometry using 678 Hz and 1000 Hz probe tones. In addition, total middle ear admittance (Y) can be broken down into the contributions of mass and stiffness (B) and conductance (G). The sensitivity and specificity of multi-frequency and multi-component tympanometry can, in some cases, exceed that of conventional 226 Hz tympanometry (Harris, Hutchinson, & Moravec, 2005).

In this chapter we discuss how to conduct and interpret multi-frequency and multi-component tympanometry. More specifically, the following tests are covered in this chapter:

- Y1000 Hz tympanometry
- B/G 678 and/or B/G1000 Hz tympanometry
- Resonant frequency evaluation

Y1000 HZ TYMPANOMETRY

Researchers have shown that for infants, Y1000 Hz tympanometry gives more reliable and valid findings than Y226 Hz tympanometry (Shanks & Shohet, 2009). That tympanometry for adults and infants differs should not be surprising considering that infants' ears differ from adults' in many ways, including immature anatomy, and at times the presence of middle ear mesenchyme. Accordingly, the American Academy of Family Practice guidelines (Rosenfeld et al., 2004) suggested the use of Y1000 Hz up to age 4 months, after which Y226 Hz is appropriate.

Procedure

The procedure is the same as for Y226 Hz tympanometry, except 1000 Hz probe tones are recommended.

Norms and Interpretation

Classification patterns have been proposed but it is often sufficient to make judgments based on Y1000 Hz tympanogram shape. Normal shape is single peaked; if one were to draw a line from the negative tail to the positive tail, that line should angle upward, and the single peak should be above the line. Abnormal shape is one peak below that line, flat and/or wide tympanograms, or multi-peaked tympanograms (Figure 11–1).

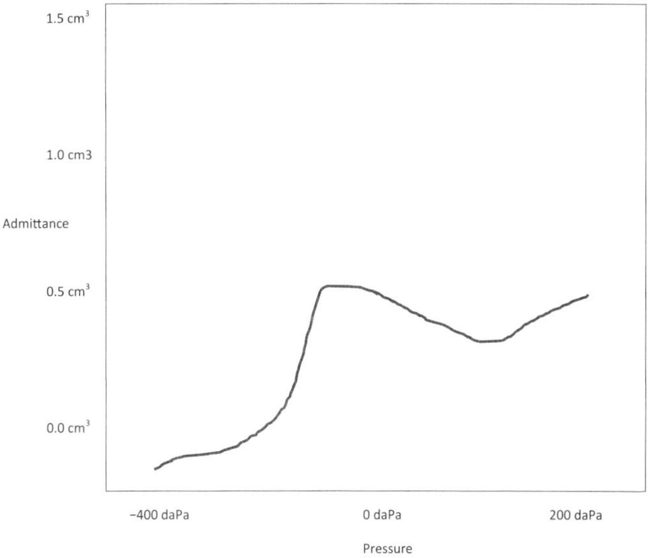

Figure 11–1. Neonate normal Y1000 Hz tympanogram.

B/G 678 AND/OR B/G 1000 HZ TYMPANOMETRY IN CHILDREN AND ADULTS

Probe Tone Frequency

For adults, Y226 Hz tympanometry provides information regarding middle-ear stiffness, just as middle-ear disorders causing stiffness can manifest as low-frequency stiffness tilt audiograms (low-frequency hearing loss). In contrast, higher frequency tympanometry, including 678 and 1000 Hz tympanometry, provides information regarding middle-ear mass characteristics (Fowler & Shanks, 2002; Lilly, 2005), just as middle ear disorders adding mass can manifest as high-frequency mass tilt audiograms (high-frequency hearing loss).

Measurement Components

In addition, admittance Y can be broken down into component parts, susceptance B and conductance G. Conductance has to do with how middle-ear friction affects admittance, whereas susceptance has to do with how middle-ear mass and stiffness affects admittance. Though the details are beyond the scope of this text, suffice it to say that in mass-controlled middle ears susceptance, admittance lags sound pressure because of middle-ear inertia. In contrast, in stiffness-controlled middle ears, susceptance admittance leads sound pressure, much as a spring initially admits energy before tightening. Therefore, mass and stiffness susceptance are in opposition, allowing for scientific plotting of admittance as a vector.

Procedure

Select desired frequency and components; for example, the Grason Stadler Tympstar can be set to test both B and G by selecting B/G. The frequency can be set either to 678 Hz or 1000 Hz. Recording Y678 and Y1000 Hz are optional.

Norms and Interpretation

Mass and stiffness tympanograms have been classified by the number of upward peaks plus the number of downward peaks (Fowler & Shanks, 2002; Vanhuyse, Creten, & Van Camp, 1975). Some of the possible shapes are shown in Figure 11–2 on a vector plot from 1B1G stiffness controlled to 5B3G mass controlled. Table 11–1 contains verbal summaries.

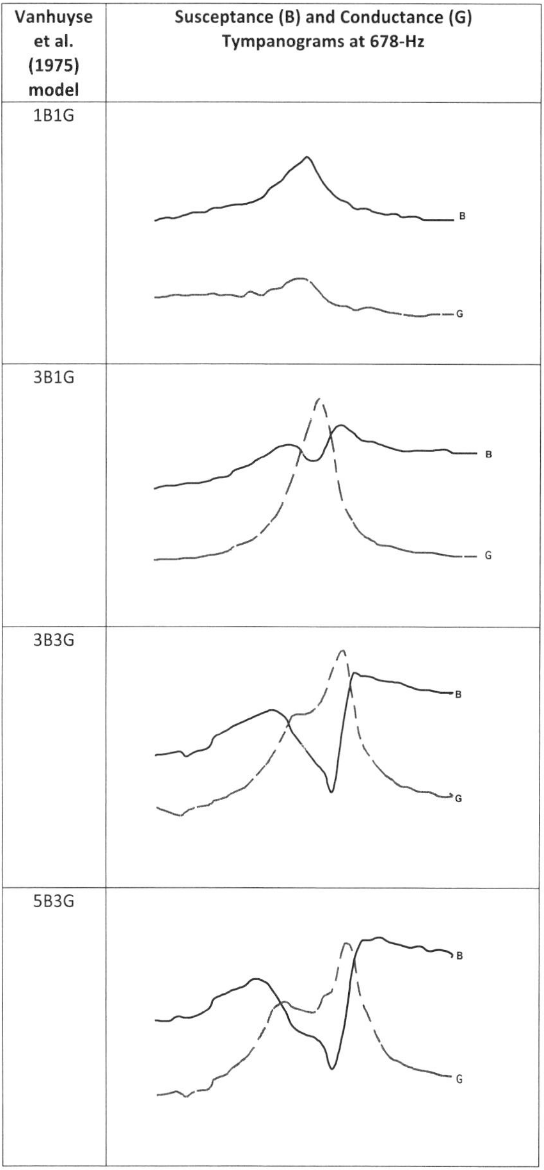

Figure 11–2. Four multicomponent tympanogram shapes. From *Acoustic immittance measures* (Page 70, Figure 5–5) by L. Hunter & N. Shahnaz, 2014, San Diego, CA: Plural Publishing, Inc. Reprinted with permission.

Table 11–1. High Frequency Y, B, and G Shapes (Vanhuyse, Creten, & Van Camp, 1975; Fowler & Shanks, 2002)

B/G Pattern	*B/G Description*	*Interpretation*
1B1G: Stiffness dominant	Both B678 and 1000 Hz and the G678 and 1000 Hz tympanograms are single-peaked. The peaks are in the positive direction (above the tympanogram tails).	Normal
1B1G narrow: Stiffness dominant	Both B678 and 1000 Hz and the G678 and 1000 Hz tympanograms are single-peaked with a narrow width. The peaks are in the positive direction (above the tympanogram tails).	Sometimes seen with ossicular fixation
3B1G: Stiffness dominant	The B678 and 1000 Hz tympanogram have three peaks; the left most peak is upward, the middle peak is downward, and the right most peak is upward. The G678 and 1000 Hz tympanogram is single peaked. All peaks are in the positive direction; that is, they are above the tympanogram tails.	Normal
3B3G or 5B3G: Mass dominant	Both the B678 and 1000 Hz and the G678 and 1000 Hz tympanograms have three or five peaks, as described above. The center B678 and 1000 Hz tympanogram peak is in the negative direction; it is below the tympanogram tails.	This indicates possible mass effect.

Table 11–1. *continued*

B/G Pattern	*B/G Description*	*Interpretation*
5B5G or 3B5G:	Variable, depending on number of peaks	Normal or tympanic membrane monomer/dimer manifests as lateral most peaks are <75daPa apart on 3-peaked tympanograms and <100daPa apart on 5-peaked tympanograms. In contrast, ossicular disarticulation manifests as lateral most peaks >75daPa on 3-peaked tympanograms and >100daPa apart on 5-peaked tympanograms
Flat with B > G	Tympanograms are flat (wide width) as with Y226 Hz tympanograms, discussed earlier in the previous chapter. B is greater (higher) than G because the middle mass, middle ear effusion, or outer ear cerumen occlusion adds middle ear susceptance.	Significant middle mass, middle ear effusion, or outer ear cerumen occlusion

continues

Table 11–1. *continued*

B/G Pattern	*B/G Description*	*Interpretation*
Flat with B < G	Tympanograms are flat (wide width) as with Y226 Hz tympanograms, discussed earlier in the previous chapter. B is lower (less than) G because pressure bypasses the middle ear through the perforation or PE tube; the middle ear cannot add susceptance.	Perforation or PE tube

Simplified clinical decision rules are offered below:

- Number of peaks rules: <5B peaks and/or <3G peaks are seen with normal middle ears (Harris, Hutchinson, & Moravec, 2005); in fact over 90% of normal middle ears show 1B1G or 3B1G patterns (Wiley, Oviatt, & Block, 1987). More peaks suggest mass affect, which can result from many disorders.
- Reliability rule: Middle ears should show no increase in the number of peaks at annual or other re-tests. Change is abnormal, even if the retest results are <5B peaks and/or <3G peaks.
- The 3B3G tympanograms with outermost maxima separated by <75 daPa is seen with normal middle ears or with monomeric/dimeric tympanic membranes.

Wider maxima separation is seen with ossicular disarticulation. Results from both monomeric/dimeric tympanic membranes and ossicular disarticulations will also show high static admittance.

- The 5B3G tympanograms with outermost maxima separated by <100 daPa is seen with normal middle ears or with monomeric/dimeric tympanic membranes. Wider maxima separation is seen with ossicular disarticulation. Results from both monomeric/dimeric tympanic membranes and ossicular disarticulations will also show high static admittance.
- Flat with B > G is seen with outer ear or middle ear occlusion.
- Flat with G < B is seen with tympanic membrane perforation or PE tube.

RESONANT FREQUENCY EVALUATION

The resonant frequency of the normal adult middle ear varies depending on measurement procedures; audiologists should consult their tympanometers manual or manufacturer for normative data.

Procedure

Procedures are equipment specific, consult your equipment manual. For example, the Grason Stadler Tympstar measures middle ear resonance using the multi-frequency procedure based on (Funasaka, Funai, & Kumakawa, 1984; Funasaka & Kumakawa,

1988) in which tympanograms are measured in 50 Hz probe tone intervals. As probe tone frequency approaches a normal middle ears' resonant frequency, tympanograms manifest peaks, and at the resonant peak the middle-most peak is neither higher nor lower than the tympanogram tails.

Norms and Interpretation

- Mass effect: Added mass might lower middle ears' resonant frequency near to or even below 800 Hz. In unilateral disorder, look also for asymmetry when comparing right and left ears. Pathologies that could add mass to the middle ear include middle ear effusion (Lai, Li, Xian, & Liu, 2008), and disarticulated ossicular chains, which can mimic added mass (Hunter & Margolis, 1992).
- Stiffness effect: Added stiffness might raise middle ears' resonant frequency near to or even above 1200 Hz. In unilateral disorder, look also for asymmetry when comparing right and left ears. Pathologies that could stiffen the middle ear include ossicular fixation (Hunter & Margolis, 1992), Eustachian tube dysfunction, and otitis media.
- Large Vestibular Aqueduct (LVA): Long-standing LVA tends to yield low resonant frequencies in the presence of stable sensory/neural hearing loss and low-frequency air-bone gaps (Bilgen, Kirkim, & Kirazli, 2009; Mimura et al., 2005; Rosowski, Songer, Nakajima, Brinsko, & Merchant, 2004; Sato, Nakashima, Lilly,

Fausti, and Ueda, 2002). The lower resonant frequency is due to LVA opening a "third window," which could lower inner ear pressure. Because the middle ear interfaces with the inner ear, the middle-ear resonance can manifest as low. Hypothetically, superior canal dehiscence could similarly manifest (Rosowski, et al., 2004).

CAVEATS

Several disorders can cause either a mass effect or a stiffness effect. Therefore it would be a mistake to expect that a multi-peak mass pattern necessarily indicates a "mass" or "growth." For example, otitis media with effusion can manifest as either a mass pattern or a stiffness pattern, perhaps depending on the amount and viscosity of the effusion. Finally, as is always true with tympanometry, different disorders might manifest with similar immittance results, and lateral pathologies obscure medial pathologies.

EXHORTATION

We find many audiologists balk at the notion of conducting multi-frequency tympanometry, even as they accept conducting many other tests at multiple frequencies, including air conduction thresholds, acoustic reflex thresholds, acoustic reflex decay, auditory brainstem response, and VNG/rotary chair. Moreover, we have heard audiologists say they would conduct tympanograms at frequencies other than 226 Hz if shown that testing at those frequencies is *better*. Evidently, only tympanometry is subject to that requirement. We urge audiologists to consider conducting high frequency tympanometry in addition to low-frequency tympanometry, not because it is better but because it is *different*; low-frequency tympanometry is more sensitive to changes in stiffness, whereas high-frequency tympanometry is more sensitive to changes in mass. The artful use of a tympanometric test battery can result in improved sensitivity and/or sensitivity.

REFERENCES

Bilgen, C., Kirkim, G., & Kirazli, T. (2009). Middle ear impedance measurements in large vestibular aqueduct syndrome. *Auris Nasus Larynx, 36*(3), 263–268. http://dx.doi.org/10.1016/j.anl.2008.07.002

Fowler, C. G., & Shanks, J. E. (2002). Tympanometry. In J. Katz (Ed.), *Handbook of clinical audiology* (5th ed., pp.175–202). Baltimore, MD: Lippincott Williams & Wilkins.

Funasaka, S., Funai, H., & Kumakawa, K. (1984). Sweep-frequency tympanometry: Its development and diagnostic value. *Audiology*, *23*, 366–379.

Funasaka, S., & Kumakawa, K. (1988). Tympanometry using a sweep-frequency probe tone and its clinical evaluation. *Audiology*, *27*, 99–108.

Harris, P.K., Hutchinson, K. M., & Moravec, J. (2005). The use of tympanometry and pneumatic otoscopy for predicting middle ear disease. *American Journal of Audiology*, *14*, 3–13.

Hunter, L. L., & Margolis, R. H. (1992). Multifrequency tympanometry. *American Journal of Audiology, 1*, 33–43. http://dx.doi.org/10.1044/1059-0889.0103.33

Lai, D., Li, W., Xian, J., & Liu, S. (2008). Multifrequency tympanometry in adults with otitis media with effusion. *European Archives of Oto-Rhino-Laryngology, 265*, 1021–1025. http://dx.doi.org/10.1007/s00405-008-0705-x

Lilly, D. (2005, April 12). The evolution of aural acoustic-immittance measurements. *The ASHA Leader, 6*, 24.

Mimura, T., Sato, E., Sugiura, M., Yoshino, T., Naganawa, S., & Nakashima, T. (2005). Hearing loss in patients with enlarged vestibular aqueduct: Air-bone gap and audiological Bing test. *International Journal of Audiology, 44*(8), 466–469.

Rosenfeld, R. M., Culpepper, L., Doyle, K., Grundfast, K. M., Hoberman, A., Kenna, M. A., . . . Yawn, B. (2004). Clinical practice guideline: Otitis media with effusion, *Otolaryngology-Head and Neck Surgery, 130*(5) S95–S118. http://dx.doi.org/10.1016/j.otohns.2004.02.002

Rosowski, J. J., Songer, J. E., Nakajima, H. H., Brinsko, K. M., & Merchant, S. N. (2004). Clinical, experimental and theoretical investigations of the effect of superior semicircular canal dehiscence on hearing mechanisms. *Otology and Neurotology, 25*(3), 323–332.

Sato, D., Nakashima, T., Lilly, D.J., Fausti, A., & Ueda, H. (2002). Tympanometric findings in patients with enlarged vestibular aqueducts. *Laryngoscope, 112,* 1642–1646.

Shanks, J., & Shohet, J. (2009). Tympanometry in clinical practice. In J. Katz (Ed.), *Handbook of clinical audiology.* (6th ed., pp. 189–221). Baltimore, MD: Lippincott Williams & Wilkins.

Vanhuyse, V., Creten, W., & Van Camp, K. (1975). On the W-notching of tympanograms. *Scandinavian Audiology, 4*(1), 45–50. http://dx.doi.org/10.3109/01050397509075014

Wiley, T. L., Oviatt, D. L., & Block, M. G. (1987). Acoustic-immittance measures in normal ears. *Journal of Speech and Hearing Research, 30*, 161–170.

12

Acoustic Reflex Evaluation for Site of Lesion

WHAT IS A REFLEX?

A reflex is an involuntary action or movement. We have hundreds of reflexes in our bodies. Examples include the pupillary light reflex involving cranial nerve II and III, the patellar reflex involving the femoral nerve, and the acoustic reflex involving cranial nerves VII and VIII.

The Acoustic Reflex

The acoustic reflex arc is bilateral; a loud sound to one ear evokes a stapedial contraction bilaterally. When the stapedial muscles contract, the result is a momentary reduction in middle ear peak admittance, which we measure with our equipment.

Acoustic Reflex Pathway

- outer, middle, inner ear on stimulated side
- VIII nerve on stimulated side
- ventral cochlear nucleus on stimulated side
- superior olivary complex and motor nuclei of VII nerves bilaterally
- VII nerves bilaterally
- stapedial branches of the VII nerve bilaterally
- stapedial muscles bilaterally

ACOUSTIC REFLEX TEST CONDITIONS

Acoustic reflex measures are made in four test conditions. Table 12–1 shows those conditions, including the presentation ear (which receives the tone), the measurement ear (in which the reflex is measured), and anatomical sites involved.

THE ACOUSTIC REFLEX THRESHOLD (ART)

The measure referred to above is the ART, which is the lowest intensity level that will evoke a reflex. For tone stimuli, ART is measured from 70 to 100 dBHL for 500 Hz to 4000 Hz pure-tones in normally hearing individuals (Newman & Sandridge, 2007).

Table 12–1. Acoustic Reflex Threshold Test Conditions, Presentation and Measurement Ears, and Anatomical Sites Involved

Test Condition	***Tone Presentation Ear***	***Acoustic Reflex Measurement Ear***	***Anatomical Sites Involved***
Right ipsilateral (also known as uncrossed)	Tone presented right	Acoustic reflex measured right	Right outer, middle, and inner ear, the right VIII nerve, related brainstem neurons, the right VII nerve, and again the right outer, and middle, ear
Left contralateral (also known as crossed)	Tone presented left	Acoustic reflex measured right	Left outer, middle, and inner ear, the left VIII nerve, related brainstem neurons, the right VII nerve, and the right outer, and middle, ear
Left ipsilateral (also known as uncrossed)	Tone presented left	Acoustic reflex measured left	Left outer, middle, and inner ear, the left VIII nerve, related brainstem neurons, the left VII nerve, and again the left outer, and middle, ear
Right contralateral (also known as crossed)	Tone presented right	Acoustic reflex measured left	Right outer, middle and inner ear, the right VIII nerve, related brainstem neurons, the left VII *nerve, and the left outer, and middle*, ear

THE ART MEASUREMENT

Instructions

Instruct the patient regarding the purpose of the task, what they will hear, and that they need not respond but instead should remain quiet and still. Assure patients that the tones will not be loud enough to cause damage.

Procedure

Use an ascending threshold search approach to avoid discomfort; start at 70 dBHL or 80 dBHL. Watch for signs of patient discomfort and consider omitting the procedure altogether for tinnitus evaluations or when hyperacusis is reported. Present one-second duration tones with 3- to 5-second rest periods between tone presentations. Changes in the peak acoustic admittance equivalent to at least .02 cm^3 likely indicate an acoustic reflex. However, this threshold should be confirmed by establishing the response again at that same intensity level or if possible by increasing 5 dB and seeing a growth of at least .02 cm^3. For safety we recommend not exceeding presentation levels of 105 dB HL.

Test Frequencies

We measure ART at 500 Hz, 1000 Hz, 2000 Hz, and 4000 Hz. We do not test 250 Hz, as low-frequency tones might interact with the Y226 Hz measurement probe tone, giving inaccurate results. Higher frequencies are omitted because many people without disorder nonetheless have abnormal high-frequency acoustic reflex thresholds.

INTERPRETATION: SEVEN RULES

Rule 1: Normal

> *Acoustic reflex thresholds in patients with normal hearing and normal middle ear function will occur between 70 and 100 dBHL.*
>
> —Newman and Sandridge, 2007, page 115

Note. They will also be at >60 dB SL

Rule 2: Conductive Disorder

> *. . . the probe ear principle states that acoustic reflexes are usually absent when there is a conductive pathology in the probe ear. In this case, the conductive pathology prevents us from being able to monitor changes in acoustic immittance at the probe tip (even though the stapedial muscle may be contracting).*
>
> —Gelfand, 2009, page 198

Rule 3: Conductive Disorder

> *. . . the stimulus ear principle states that a conductive disorder in the stimulus ear reduces the stimulus level reaching the cochlea by the amount of the air-bone gap. As a result the*

ART is elevated by the amount of the air-bone gap and will be absent if it is elevated beyond the maximum available stimulus level.

—Gelfand, 2009, page 198

Rule 4: Cochlear Pathology

. . . the acoustic reflex is elicited at sensation levels of less than 60 dB[SL] in ears with cochlear lesions . . . there is a 90% likelihood of observing the acoustic reflex as long as the cochlear hearing loss is less than 60 dB[HL]. As the cochlear loss increases above 60 dB[HL], chances of observing the reflex decreases.

—Northern, Gabbard and Kinder, 1985, page 482

Same rule, different authors:

Mild cochlear hearing loss has little effect on acoustic reflex thresholds. In contrast, reflexes probably will be absent when audiometric thresholds exceed 80 dBHL. When the cochlear hearing loss is <80 dBHL, acoustic reflex thresholds may be present but at reduced sensation levels.

—Newman and Sandridge, 2007, page 115

Rule 5: VIII Nerve Pathology

When stimulating an ear with VIII nerve pathology, *The presence of acoustic reflexes in eighth nerve disorders is the exception rather than the rule as shown by many authors . . .*

—Northern et al., 1985, page 484

Rule 6: VII Nerve Pathology

> *Acoustic reflexes are abnormal or absent when the probe is placed in the ear with facial nerve paralysis. Acoustic reflex responses are obtained only if the site of lesion is central to the innervation of the stapes muscle.*
>
> —Newman and Sandridge, 2007, page 116

Same rule with more precise site of lesion evaluation:

> *If the acoustic reflex is present at normal [levels], the localization of pathology is likely distal to the stapedius branch of the nerve. If reflexes are absent [or] present but elevated, the disorder is likely proximal to the nerve.*
>
> —Northern et al., 1985, page 485

Rule 7: Intra-Axial (Brainstem) Pathology

> *The absence of contralateral acoustic reflexes, with ipsilateral acoustic reflexes intact, may be seen in patients with. . . brainstem pathology. . . in the area of the crossed brainstem pathways while the uncrossed pathways remain intact.*
>
> —Northern et al., 1985, page 485

Clinician Cheat Sheet

- Conductive hearing losses cause elevated or absent reflexes.
- Outer hair cell disorder results in reflexes at normal dB HL but low dB SL.

- Inner hair cell disorder causes elevated or absent reflexes.
- VII, VIII, and low to mid-brainstem disorder causes elevated or absent reflexes.

ACOUSTIC REFLEX TRACE ANOMALIES (GELFAND, 2002)

- Opposite phase at onset and offset: possible stapes fixation " . . . attributed to elasticity changes in the stapes and annular ligament that are associated with the partial fixation of the footplate at the oval window" (page 209).
- Opposite phase at onset only: associated with a momentary decoupling of the interface between stapes and cochlea fluids
- During ipsilateral testing, constructive or destructive interference of probe and stimuli tones in the ear canal can cause artificially enhanced or diminished reflex traces.

ACOUSTIC REFLEX DECAY (ADAPTATION)

This supra reflex-threshold test is used to measure the magnitude of the acoustic reflex over time, thus allowing the audiologists to assess adaptation, the inability of VIII nerve neurons to recover after firing. Adaptation can be affected (lengthened) by VII or VIII nerve pathology.

Procedure

Test at 500 Hz and 1000 Hz if possible; the test can only safely be conducted if an ART was measured at 95 dB HL or less. Test contralaterally if possible, if not attempt ipsilaterally testing (Martin & Clark, 2015). Present a tone for 10 seconds at 10 dB above the previously measured ART. Monitor acoustic reflex amplitude.

Interpretation

Retrocochlear pathology is suspected if the reflex decays in magnitude by 50% at either test frequency within 10 seconds. Sensitivity increases if decay occurs in 5 seconds or less.

REFERENCES

Gelfand, S. A. (2002). The acoustic reflex. In J. Katz (Ed.), *Handbook of clinical audiology* (5th ed., pp. 205–221). Baltimore, MD: Lippincott Williams & Wilkins.

Gelfand, S. A. (2009). The acoustic reflex. In J. Katz (Ed.), *Handbook of clinical audiology* (5th ed., pp. 189–221). Baltimore, MD: Lippincott Williams & Wilkins.

Martin, F. N., & Clark, J. G. (2015). *Introduction to audiology* (12th ed.). Boston, MA: Pearson.

Newman, C. W., & Sandridge, S. A. (2007). Diagnostic audiology. In G. B. Hughes & M. L. Pensak (Eds.), *Clinical otology* (3rd ed., pp. 109–120). New York, NY: Thieme.

Northern, J. L., Gabbard, S. A., & Kinder, D. L. (1985). The acoustic reflex. In J. Katz (Ed.), *Handbook of clinical audiology* (3rd ed. pp. 476–495). Baltimore, MD: Lippincott Williams & Wilkins.

13

Hearing Threshold Estimation by Acoustic Reflex Threshold (ART)

OVERVIEW

Acoustic reflexes are evoked by loud sounds. Researchers have studied the relationship between acoustic reflex thresholds and hearing thresholds and have proposed ways to use the former to predict the latter. Though the resulting predictions are imperfect, they might be useful as a screening tool, especially with patients unwilling or unable to cooperate in behavioral testing. Four methods will be discussed here:

1. Broadband noise (BBN) acoustic reflex threshold (ART) screening
2. Sensitivity prediction by acoustic reflex (SPAR) and a SPAR shortcut
3. The 10th percentile table
4. ART at audible level rule

BBN SCREENING TOOL

Procedure

Start a BBN ART search at 60 dB SPL because BBN stimulates more hair cells and neurons than pure-tones do, and thus BBN tend to evoke ART at lower intensity levels than seen with pure-tones. Changes in the peak acoustic admittance equivalent to at least .02 cm^3 likely indicate an acoustic reflex. However, this threshold should be confirmed by establishing the response again at that same intensity level or if possible by increasing 5 dB and seeing a growth of at least .02 cm^3. For safety we recommend not exceeding presentation levels of 90 dB SPL.

Interpretation

A BBN ART at ≤85 dB SPL suggests three-frequency pure-tone average (PTA) ≤40, that is, no worse than a mild PTA hearing loss. This screening tool has a sensitivity of 97% and specificity of 87% (Keith, 1977).

SPAR

Sensitivity Prediction by Acoustic Reflexes (SPAR; Jerger, Burney, Mauldin, & Crump, 1974; Niemeyer & Sesterhenn, 1974) is based on comparing the BBN ART to tone evoked ART at 500 Hz, 1000 Hz, and 2000 Hz. ART differences for BBN and tones have been documented for normally hearing listeners and for listeners with various degrees of hearing loss; this allows hearing sensitivity prediction.

Procedure

Obtain the following ART and make the following calculations:

A. = 500 Hz ART in dB HL. Add 13 dB to convert to dB SPL
B. = 1000 Hz ART in dB HL. Add 7 dB to convert to dB SPL
C. = 2000 Hz ART in dB HL. Add 11 dB to convert to dB SPL
D. = (A + B + C) ÷ 3
E. = Lowest of A, B, and C
F. = BBN reflex threshold (no dB SPL conversion needed)
G. = D − F
H. = A − F
I. = E − F
J. = (G + H + I) ÷ 3

SPAR Interpretation

- J ≥20 and BBN at *any* level, predicts WNL
- J 15 to 19 and BBN ≤80, predicts WNL
- J 15 to 19 and BBN >80, predicts mild-mod loss
- J 10 to 14 and BBN any level, predicts mild-mod loss
- J <10 and BBN ≤89, predicts severe loss
- J <10 and BBN >89, predicts profound loss

Example using the first author's ART

A. = 95 dB HL + 13 = 108 dB SPL
B. = 85 dB HL + 7 = 92 dB SPL
C. = 95 dB HL + 11= 106 dB SPL

D. = (A+B+C)/3 = 102 dB SPL
E. = Lowest of A, B, and C = 92 dB SPL
F. = BBN reflex = 80 dB SPL
G. = D − F = 102 − 80 = 22
H. = A − F = 108 − 80 = 28
I. = E − F = 92 − 80 = 12
J. = (G+H+I) ÷ 3
= 22 + 28 + 12 ÷ 3
= 62 ÷ 3
= 20.67, which predicts normal hearing, no worse than a mild hearing loss in the 500- to 2000-Hz range

Spar Sensitivity (Jerger, Hayes, Anthony, & Mauldin, 1978)

- 100% of those predicted to have normal hearing sensitivity showed normal hearing sensitivity on their audiograms (100% specificity).
- 85% of those predicted to have severe hearing loss showed severe hearing loss on their audiograms (85% sensitivity for severe or greater loss).
- 54% of those predicted to have moderate hearing loss showed moderate hearing loss on their audiograms (54% sensitivity for moderate loss).

MARTIN AND CLARK (2015) SPAR SHORTCUT

A. = 500 Hz ART converted from dB HL to dB SPL (add 13)
B. = 1000 Hz ART converted from dB HL to dB SPL (add 7)

C. = 2000 Hz ART converted from dB HL to dB SPL (add 11)
D. = BBN reflex
E. = (A+B+C) ÷ 3
F. E − BBN ART

Interpretation (Martin & Clark, 2015, p. 378)

- Normal = "about 25 dB"
- Mild to moderate losses "show only a 10 to 20 dB difference"
- Moderately severe losses "show less than 10 dB difference"
- Severe losses "show no acoustic reflexes"

Example using the first author's ART
A. = 95 dB HL + 13 = 108 dB SPL
B. = 85 dB HL + 7 = 92 dB SPL
C. = 95 dB HL + 11= 106 dB SPL
D. BBN reflex = 80 dB SPL
E. = (A+B+C) ÷ 3 = 102 dBS PL
F. 102 − 80 = 22 dB SPL which predicts normal hearing

THE 10TH PERCENTILE: ANOTHER USEFUL TOOL FOR PSEUDOHYPOACUSIS

The 10th percentile cutoffs in Table 13–1 (Gelfand, 2002, p. 228) shows the lowest ART that can be accepted without suspicion for functional hearing loss. For example, a patient with a 500 Hz audiogram threshold of 80 dB HL would have inner hair cell damage and thus would be unlikely to have an ART less than 100 dB HL. Lower intensity ART for

Table 13–1. The Lowest Acoustic Reflex Thresholds that Can Be Accepted Without Suspicion for Functional Hearing Loss (Gelfand, 2002, p. 228)

Audiogram Thresholds (dB HL)	*500 Hz*	*1000 Hz*	*2000 Hz*
<60 dB HL	Not recommended	Not recommended	Not recommended
60 dB HL	85 dB HL reflex	85 dB HL reflex	85 dB HL reflex
65 dB HL	90 dB HL reflex	90 dB HL reflex	90 dB HL reflex
70 dB HL	95 dB HL reflex	95 dB HL reflex	90 dB HL reflex
75 dB HL	95 dB HL reflex	95 dB HL reflex	95 dB HL reflex
80 dB HL	100 dB HL reflex	100 dB HL reflex	100 dB HL reflex
85 dB HL	100 dB HL reflex	100 dB HL reflex	110 dB HL reflex
≥90	10 dB SL reflex	10 dB SL reflex	10 dB SL reflex

this patient would be inconsistent with inner hair cell damage, suggesting the 80-dB HL audiogram threshold to be invalid.

ART AT INAUDIBLE LEVELS

As shown in Table 13–1, acoustic reflex thresholds are unlikely to be obtained at very low dB SL. Extending the concept, acoustic reflex thresholds cannot be obtained at inaudible levels. Therefore, if ARTs are measured below audiogram thresholds, pseudohypoacusis is likely.

REFERENCES

Gelfand, S. A. (2002). The acoustic reflex. In J. Katz (Ed.), *Handbook of clinical audiology* (6th ed., pp. 205–232). Baltimore, MD: Lippincott Williams & Wilkins.

Jerger, J., Burney, P., Mauldin, L., & Crump, B. (1974). Predicting hearing loss from the acoustic reflex. *Journal of Speech and Hearing Disorders, 39,* 11–22. http://dx.doi.org/10.1044/jshd.3901.11

Jerger, J. F., Hayes, D., Anthony, L., & Mauldin, L. (1978). Factors influencing prediction of hearing levels from the acoustic reflex. *Monographs in Contemporary Audiology, 1*, 1–20.

Keith, R. W. (1977). An evaluation of predicting hearing loss from acoustic reflex. *Archives of Otolaryngology, 103*(7). 419–424. http://dx.doi.org/10.1001/archotol.1977.00780240077012

Martin, F. N. (1994). *Introduction to audiology* (5th ed.). Boston, MA: Allyn & Bacon.

Martin, F. N., & Clark, J. G. (2015). *Introduction to audiology* (12th ed.). Boston, MA: Pearson.

Niemeyer, W., & Sesterhenn, G. (1974). Calculating the hearing threshold from the stapedius reflex threshold for different sound stimuli. *Audiology, 13*(5), 421–427. http://dx.doi.org/10.3109/00206097409071701

14 Eustachian Tube and Vascular Anomalies Tests

OVERVIEW

The Eustachian tube serves to aerate the middle ear; when it is functionally or structurally blocked, aeration cannot occur. Functional blockage can occur by collapse of a compliant cartilaginous portion in children or insufficient tensor veli palatini muscles, whereas structural blockage can be caused by adenoid enlargement, inflammation, edema, mucous, and, rarely, tumors. According to the ex vaccuo theory, Eustachian tube dysfunction (ETD) results in negative middle ear pressure because air in the middle ear space is absorbed by cells in the walls of the middle ear (Sade & Luntz, 1992), though this is debated (Hergils & Magnuson, 1988). It is also possible that sucking, as an adult would do on a cigarette or a child would do on a bottle or pacifier, could create a negative oral pressure and draw air from the middle ear through the Eustachian tube (Ibrahim & Fatt-hi, 1983).

Regardless of etiology or process, negative middle ear pressure is a partial vacuum that can draw inter and intracellular fluids from the middle ear (ME) walls. This effusion can cause conductive hearing loss. The Y226 Hz pressure peak, discussed in an earlier chapter, is an indirect test of Eustachian tube function. A normal pressure peak suggests normal Eustachian tube functioning, whereas a negative pressure peak suggests ETD. In this chapter we review direct Eustachian tube tests with intact tympanic membranes (Valsalva, Toynbee, inflation, and deflation) and perforated tympanic membranes (inflation and deflation). We also discuss testing for patulous (patent) Eustachian tubes.

Finally, we discuss the use of tympanometers to differentially diagnose ETD from vascular anomalies. Causes of vascular anomaly include, but are not limited to, blood vessel abnormalities in the tympanic membrane, or middle ear pathology, for example, glomus tumor. Such patients might present with pulsatile tinnitus consistent with heartbeat.

EUSTACHIAN TUBE TESTS WITH INTACT TYMPANIC MEMBRANES

Valsalva Procedure (Reidel, Wiley, & Block, 1987)

- Obtain a baseline Y226 Hz tympanogram.
- Ask the patient to perform the Valsalva maneuver; the patient must close his/her mouth, pinch the nares closed, and attempt to inflate the middle ear through forced expiration. The patient may then release the nares but must refrain from further

mandibular movement or swallowing until testing is completed.

- Obtain a post-Valsalva Y226 Hz tympanogram.
- Post-test: recommend drinking water and swallowing to open the Eustachian tubes to return middle ear pressure to normal.

Valsalva Interpretation

The Valsalva maneuver normally forces air up the Eustachian tube and into the middle ear space, thus shifting middle ear pressure in the positive direction. Accordingly, Reidel et al. (1987) reported 95% Valsalva shift confidence limits of 47 to 79 daPa (Figure 14–1). Shifts of this magnitude suggest normal Eustachian tube functioning.

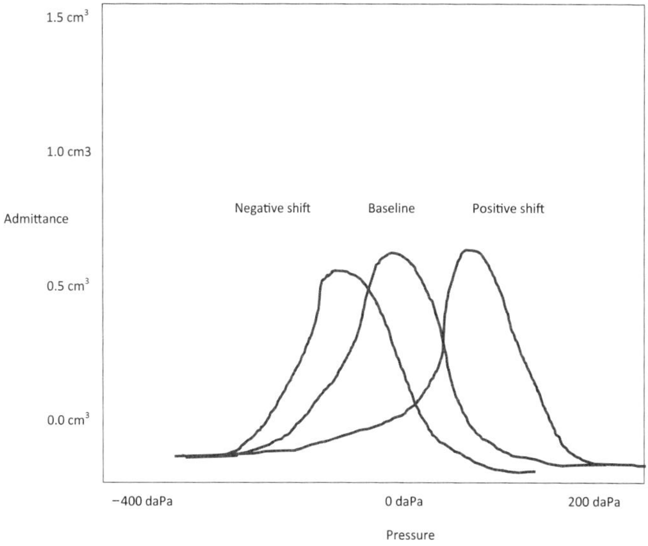

Figure 14–1. Example of a positive shift from Valsalva or inflation and a negative shift from Toynbee or deflation.

Toynbee Procedure (Reidel et al., 1987)

- Obtain a baseline Y226 Hz tympanogram.
- Ask the patient to perform the Toynbee maneuver; patient must close his/her mouth, pinch the nares closed, and swallow. The patient may then release the nares but must refrain from further mandibular movement or swallowing until testing is completed.
- Obtain a post-Toynbee Y226 Hz tympanogram.
- Post-test: recommend drinking water and swallowing to return middle ear pressure to normal.

Toynbee Interpretation

The Toynbee maneuver normally creates a negative oral pressure that draws air down the Eustachian tube and out of the middle ear space, thus shifting middle ear pressure in the negative direction. Accordingly, Reidel et al. (1987) reported 95% Toynbee confidence limits of −4 to −26 daPa (see Figure 14–1). Shifts of this magnitude suggest normal Eustachian tube functioning.

Inflation Procedure (Reidel et al., 1987)

- Obtain a baseline Y226 Hz tympanogram.
- The ear canal is inflated by manually increasing pressure to +400 daPa. The patient is then asked to swallow several times with water.
- The applied ear-canal pressure is returned to 0 daPa, and a test Y226 Hz tympanogram is obtained.

- Post-test: recommend drinking water and swallowing to return middle ear pressure to normal; this can be confirmed with a post-test Y226 Hz tympanogram.

Inflation Interpretation

Inflating the ear canal normally forces air down the Eustachian tube and out of the middle ear space, thus shifting middle ear pressure in the negative direction. Said differently, inflating the ear canal *deflates* the middle ear. Accordingly Reidel et al. (1987) reported 95% confidence limit of −8 to −13 daPa (see Figure 14–1). Grason Stadler Instruments (GSI personal communication) agrees on the negative direction of the shift but differs in amount: −15 to −20 daPa is their normal range. Shifts of these magnitudes suggest normal Eustachian tube functioning.

Deflation Procedure (Reidel et al., 1987)

- Obtain a baseline Y226 Hz tympanogram
- The ear canal is deflated pressure by manually decreasing pressure to −400 daPa. The patient is then asked to swallow several times with water.
- The applied ear-canal pressure is returned to 0 daPa, and a test Y226 Hz tympanogram is obtained.
- Post-test: recommend drinking water and swallowing to return middle ear pressure to normal; this can be confirmed with a post-test Y226 Hz tympanogram.

Deflation Interpretation

Deflating the ear canal normally draws air up the Eustachian tube and into the middle ear space, thus shifting middle ear pressure in the positive direction. Said differently, deflating the ear canal *inflates* the middle ear. Accordingly Reidel et al. (1987) reported 95% deflation confidence limits of 12 to 18 daPa (see Figure 14–1). Grason Stadler Instruments (GSI, personal communication) agrees on the positive direction of the shift but differs in amount: 15 to 20 daPa is their normal range. Shifts of these magnitudes suggest normal Eustachian tube functioning.

RAMIFICATIONS OF ABNORMAL EUSTACHIAN TUBE TESTS WITH INTACT TYMPANIC MEMBRANES

If an abnormal finding is obtained, ETD is possible. If this is the only abnormal finding, consider educating the patient on Eustachian tube functioning and monitoring. If symptoms persist or worsen, audiologists can refer for a medical evaluation. Of course, if there are other abnormal test findings audiologists must act accordingly.

WHICH TEST IS BEST?

Of the above tests for patients with intact tympanic membranes, Reidel et al. (1987) favored Valsalva, whereas Hunter and Sanford (2015) wrote that Toynbee is considered more reliable than the Valsalva test.

EUSTACHIAN TUBE TESTS WITH PERFORATED TYMPANIC MEMBRANES

Inflation Procedure

- Manually increase pressure to +200 daPa or until the Eustachian tube is forced open and pressure is equalized to 0 daPa.
- If pressure is not equalized at +200 daPa ask the patient to drink water and swallow several times.

Inflation Interpretation

Lack of pressure equalization suggests ETD.

Deflation Procedure

- Manually decrease pressure −400 daPa or until the Eustachian tube is forced open and pressure is equalized to 0 daPa.
- If pressure is not equalized at −400 daPa, ask the patient to drink water and swallow several times.

Deflation Interpretation

Lack of pressure equalization suggests ETD.

RAMIFICATIONS OF ABNORMAL EUSTACHIAN TUBE TESTS WITH PERFORATED TYMPANIC MEMBRANES

Patients with perforated tympanic membranes should follow the recommendations of a physician; in fact, we recommend such testing only when requested by a physician.

TESTS FOR PATENT (PATULOUS) EUSTACHIAN TUBES

Patent Eustachian Tube Test Procedure: Option 1

Place the probe in the ear on the side suspected of having a patent Eustachian tube; do not place the contralateral earphone in either ear. Run a trace in contralateral acoustic reflex decay mode in the following five conditions:

1. The patient breathes through the mouth
2. The patient breathes through the nose
3. The patient breathes through the mouth with the right nostril closed
4. The patient breathes through the mouth with the left nostril closed
5. The patient holds his or her breath

Patent Eustachian Tube Test Procedure: Option 2

Place the probe in the ear on the side suspected of having a patent Eustachian tube. Select manual mode tympanometry and slowly adjust the pressure to peak static admittance. Observe static admittance in the above five conditions.

Interpretation

Patent Eustachian tubes, which might occur after significant weight loss, can cause airflow through a patent Eustachian tube and move the tympanic membrane. Breathing-related movement of the tympanic membrane can be measured with our equipment. Such patients might also report audition of breathing and/or chewing. According to McGrath and Michaelides (2011):

- Fluctuations >0.07 cm^3 suggest a patent Eustachian tube, especially when fluctuations coincide with patient breathing
- Fluctuations should disappear or diminish to <0.07 cm^3 when holding breath.

TEST FOR BLOOD VESSEL ABNORMALITIES

Blood Vessel Abnormalities Procedure

- Use one of the Eustachian tube patency test procedures described above; we recommend Option 1.

Interpretation

Blood vessel abnormalities can move the tympanic membrane with rhythmic pulses, which can be measured with our equipment. Blood vessel abnormalities could include tortuous blood vessels in the tympanic membrane or middle ear neoplasms, such as glomus tumors impinging on the ossicular chain. Patients with blood vessel abnormalities might present with pulsatile tinnitus consistent with heartbeat. According to McGrath and Michaelides (2011):

- Fluctuations <0.07 cm^3 and consistent with heartbeat suggests blood vessel abnormality.
- Fluctuations should not disappear or diminish when holding breath.

REFERENCES

Hergils L., & Magnuson B. (1988). Regulation of negative middle ear pressure without tubal opening. *Archives of Otolaryngology-Head Neck Surg*, *114*(12), 1442–1444.

Hunter, L. L., & Sanford, C. A. (2015). Tympanometry and wideband acoustic immittance. In J. Katz, M. Chasin, K. English, L. Hood, & K. Tillery (Eds.), *Handbook of clinical audiology* (7th ed., pp. 137–164). Philadelphia, PA: Wolters Kluwer.

Ibrahim A.S. & Fatt-hi A.S. (1983). Cigarette smoking and hearing loss. *American Cancer Society Journal*, *2*(2), 31–33.

McGrath, A. P., & Michaelides, E. M. (2011). Use of middle ear immittance testing in the evaluation of patulous eustachian tube. *Journal of the American Academy of Audiology*, *22*(4), 201–207.

Riedel, C. L., Wiley, T.L., & Block, M.G. (1987). Tympanometric measures of Eustachian tube function. *Journal of Speech and Hearing Research*, *30*, 207–214. http://dx.doi.org/10.1044/jshr.3002.207

Sade, J., & Luntz, M. (1992). Middle ear gases. *Acta Oto-Rhino-Laryngologica Belgica*, *46*(4), 355–360.

15

Wideband Acoustic Immittance

OVERVIEW

Wideband Acoustic Immittance (WAI) is used to measure reflected sound power, given as the percent of reflected power divided by incident power. The incident power is broad frequency "chirps" or multiple tones across frequencies. The reflected power is off the middle ear, and it is dictated by middle ear resonance. For patients with normal middle ear resonance the sound power reflectance will be lowest in roughly the 1500 to 4000 Hz range (Figure 15–1). WAI has shown promise as a tool to assess middle ear status (Feeney et al., 2013). Other WAI measures include absorbance (the reciprocal of reflectance) given in percentage or transformed to a logarithmical scale.

PROCEDURE

The procedures for WAI are equipment-specific, involving a calibration procedure in calibration

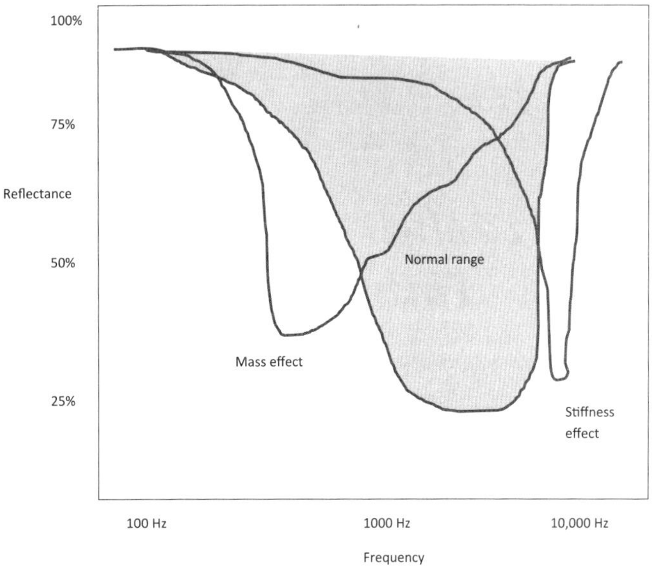

Figure 15–1. Example range of normal power reflectance, mass effect, and stiffness effect.

cavities (Allen, Jeng, & Levitt, 2005; Feeney, Grant, & Marryott, 2003). Importantly, WAI can be conducted without a hermetic seal, making it an attractive option for patients in whom a seal cannot be obtained. This option is credible in view of evidence that WAI and tympanometry correlates significantly (Schairer, Morrison, Szewczyk, & Fowler, 2011). This also suggests that WAI can be used as a cross-check of tympanometric results.

Interpretation

There are three disorders for which WAI might be of special help to audiologists for differential diagnosis; stapedial fixation, ossicular discontinuity, and superior semicircular canal dehiscence (Nakajima et al., 2012). These three conditions present similarly with audiogram air-bone gaps, an intact tympanic membrane, and a normally aerated middle ear (normal tympanogram pressure peak), but their WAI patterns are distinct (Nakajima et al., 2012).

Other disorders can affect WAI test results including otitis media with effusion, tympanic membrane monomer/dimer, and tympanic membrane perforations. Middle-ear disorders can have a stiffening effect and shift middle ear resonance to higher frequencies, or a mass effect and shift middle ear resonance to lower frequencies. Third-window, inner ear disorders affect inner ear resonance, which can be reflected in WAI measures because the middle and inner ears are coupled.

Interpretation Patterns *(see Figure 15–1)*

- Normal reflectance has a single trough of lesser reflectance (greater absorbance) in roughly the 1500 to 4000 Hz range.
- Otosclerosis also tends to shift the reflectance trough to the higher test frequencies reflecting a stiffening effect of the middle ear (Feeney et al., 2003).
- Ossicular disarticulations, tympanic membrane monomer/dimer, and tympanic membrane perforations often cause multiple reflectance troughs, with the greatest trough shifted to the lower test frequencies indicating a lower middle ear resonance (Allen, Jeng, & Levitt, 2005; Feeney et al., 2003) suggesting a mass effect.
- Superior Semicircular Canal Dehiscence power reflectance can appear somewhat normal, but with less reflectance at 1000 Hz

(Nakajima et al., 2012) or 2000 to 3000 Hz (Feeney et al., 2003).

- Otitis media can shift the sound-power reflectance trough to the higher test frequencies, reflecting a stiffening effect of the middle ear (Allen et al., 2005; Feeney et al., 2003). More viscous effusion can shift the peak to a lower frequency or result in a flat tracing.

CURRENT STATUS AND FUTURE TRENDS

Current Status

WAI is currently not widely used. The ASHA (1996) reviewed the evidence and declared WAI an inappropriate procedure for middle ear screening; they recommended otoscopy and tympanometric ear canal volume, static admittance, and width. Similarly, the American Academy of Pediatrics, American Academy of Family Physicians, and the American Academy of Otolaryngology-Head and Neck Surgery guidelines recommended otoscopy, pneumatic otoscopy and optional tympanogram confirmation (Rosenfeld et al., 2004).

Future Trends

The future of WAI is absorbance measures with pressure sweeps, so called, 3D wideband tympanometry. This test could be more sensitive than traditional tympanometry for otitis media, otosclerosis, and ossicular discontinuity (Hunter, 2013). Acoustic reflexes might also be measured with this equipment; thus WAI might one day replace traditional immittance in routine evaluation.

REFERENCES

Allen, J. B., Jeng, P. S., Levitt, H. (2005). Evaluation of human middle ear function via an acoustic power assessment. *Journal of Rehabilitation Research & Development, 42*(4), 63–78.

American Speech-Language Hearing Association. (1996). *Guidelines for audiologic screening.* Rockville, MD: Author. Available at http://www.asha.com/policy

Feeney, M. P., Grant, I. L., & Marryott, L. P. (2003). Wideband energy reflectance measurements in adults with middle-ear disorders. *Journal of Speech Language and Hearing Research, 46*, 901–911.

Feeney, M. P., Hunter, L. L., Kei, J., Lilly, D. J., Margolis, R. H., Nakajima, H. H., . . . Voss, S. E. (2013). Consensus statement: Eriksholm workshop on wideband absorbance measures of the middle ear. *Ear and Hearing, 34*, 78s–79s.

Hunter, L. (2013). 20Q: Acoustic immittance—what still works & what's new. *AudiologyOnline*. Retrieved from http://www.audiologyonline.com

Nakajima, H. H., Pisano, D. V., Roosli, C., Hamade, M. A., Merchant, G. R., Mahfoud, L., . . . Merchant, S. N. (2012). Comparison of ear-canal reflectance and umbo velocity in patients with conductive hearing loss: A preliminary study. *Ear and Hearing, 33*(1), 35–43. http://dx.doi.org/10.1097/AUD.0b013e31822ccva0

Rosenfeld, R. M., Culpepper, L., Doyle, K., Grundfast, K. M., Hoberman, A., Kenna, M. A., . . . Yawn, B. (2004). Clinical practice guideline: Otitis media with effusion. *Otolaryngology-Head and Neck Surgery, 130*(5) S95–S118. http://dx.doi.org/10.1016/j.otohns.2004.02.00

Schairer, K. S. Morrison, B; Szewczyk, E, & Fowler, C. G. (2011). Relationships among standard and wideband measures of middle ear function and distortion product otoacoustic emissions. *Journal of the American Academy of Audiology, 22*(5), 253–264.

16

Otoacoustic Emissions

OVERVIEW

Otoacoustic emissions (OAE) are sound waves originating within the cochlea that are emitted through the middle ear and in turn into the ear canal. OAE are the result of nonlinear outer hair cell (OHC) activity, which creates harmonics and distortions at frequencies not present in the signal input (Kemp, 2003). Thus, we evoke and measure OAE to assess OHC. Neither inner hair cells (IHC) nor neurons play a role in OAE production. Occlusive outer ear and middle ear disorder must be ruled out prior to OAE testing because either might block stimuli from entering the cochlea and OAE from exiting the cochlea.

We most commonly assess distortion product OAE and transient evoked OAE. The cochlear mechanics of each are complex. A full discussion is beyond our scope, but each is addressed briefly below.

DPOAE Overview

The 2f1-f2 intermodulation distortion frequency is one distortion frequency created within a normal cochlea. It is the result of the interaction of the traveling basilar membrane waves created by two tones at different frequencies delivered to the ear simultaneously. The lower frequency tone is called frequency "1," or "f1" for short, and the higher frequency tone is called "f2." For example, suppose we deliver an f1 tone of 1641 Hz and an f2 tone of 2016 Hz. Each will cause a basilar membrane traveling wave, and because the tones are close in frequency, the two traveling wave peaks will overlap. Resulting nonlinear hair cell activity will create an intermodulation distortion frequency of 1266 Hz, which can be calculated as 2 × 1641 Hz – 2016 Hz. That newly created sound wave will travel toward the oval window, which, in turn, will vibrate the middle ear including the tympanic membrane. Finally, the tympanic membrane will act as a loudspeaker diaphragm to vibrate air molecules in the ear canal. This intermodulation distortion OAE is commonly called the distortion product OAE, or DPOAE for short.

Transient-Evoked OAE (TEOAE) Overview

When transient stimuli, such as clicks are used, energy across many frequencies is delivered to the ear. Resulting intermodulation distortions are evoked (Withnell & Yates, 1998) and are, in turn, measured as OAE. Computer fast Fourier transform analysis will reveal the frequencies present in the OAE. This is the transient-evoked OAE, or TEOAE for short.

DPOAE EVALUATION

- The probe directs f1 and f2 tones of various frequencies into the ear canal. The frequency ratio of any two-tone presentation is 1.2 to 1 and the intensities of the two tones are typically 65 dB SPL and 55 dB SPL, respectively; all this is pre-programmed and delivered with a single command. A microphone in the probe transduces OAEs for computer analysis.
- The frequencies of f1 and f2 are varied in order to test different places along the tonotopically arranged basilar membrane. DPOAE arise from the place where the two tones' traveling wave peaks overlap; thus the OHC *at that place* are assessed. That place is apical to the place associated with f2 (Hall, 2000). The place can be more precisely calculated as the geometric mean frequency of f1 and f2, that is, the square root of f1 × f2. Fortunately, this is calculated by our equipment and provided on screen and in the printout.

Interpretation

- DPOAE are judged to be normal, low-amplitude, or absent, depending on their absolute intensity, intensity relative to ambient noise, and test-retest reliability. Computers offer normative DPOAE data to help audiologists make these judgments. Hall and Mueller (1997) proposed the following criteria to evaluate DPOAE presence or absence:

- DPOAE amplitude >−10 dB SPL
- DPOAE-NF >5 dB SPL
- DPOAE replicable ±5 dB SPL

When DPOAE are present at normal levels, expect normal hearing sensitivity. Specifically, expect audiometric thresholds of 15 or better dB, depending on the integrity of IHC and/or neurons. When DPOAE are low-amplitude at a given geometric mean frequency, expect the precipitating OHC disorder to cause hearing loss at and/or near that frequency. Specifically, expect audiometric thresholds of 15 to 30 dB, poorer depending on the integrity of IHC and/or neurons. When DPOAE are absent at a given geometric mean frequency, expect the precipitating OHC disorder to cause hearing loss at and/or near that frequency. Specifically, expect audiometric thresholds of 30 dB or poorer depending on the degree of OHC dysfunction and the integrity of IHC and/or neurons.

An example of DPOAE data for a patient with a high-frequency hearing loss is shown in Table 16–1, with the presence or absence of OAE decided according to the Hall and Mueller (1997) criteria (replication not included). Figure 16–1 shows an example of patient data plotted on a graph.

Caveat

The cochlear mechanics of OAE are more complex than described above, and involve nonlinear distortions and linear coherent reflections, which might result in emissions that may be in phase, and constructively interfere or be out of phase and destructively interfere. As a result, the OAE might include

Table 16–1. Example of distortion product otoacoustic emissions (DPOAE) data for a patient with a high-frequency hearing loss, with presence/absence decided according to the Hall and Mueller (1997) criteria

Geometric Mean Hz	*DPOAE (dB SPL)*	*Noise Floor (dB SPL)*	*DPOAE-NF*	*Replicable*	*Result*
7253	–13.5	–23.9	10.4	No	Absent
5130	–3.6	–11.9	8.3	Yes	Present
3616	1.9	–14.9	16.8	Yes	Present
2589	–2.2	–9.6	10.6	Yes	Present
1818	2.2	–9.6	11.8	Yes	Present

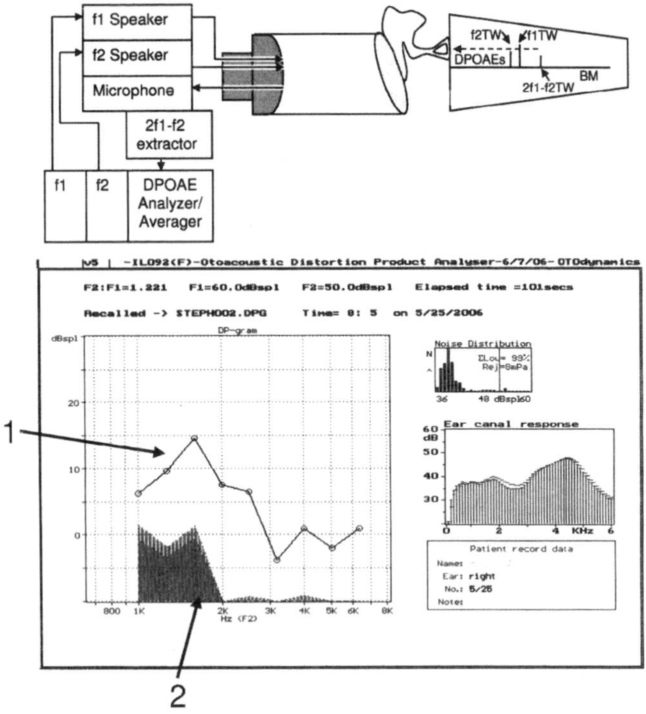

Figure 16–1. *Top:* Diagram of DPOAE apparatus showing a speaker for each of two stimuli pure-tones and a microphone to allow for analysis. *Bottom:* 1) Example data showing DPOAE (*circles*), will all > −10 dB SPL. 2) The noise floor (*shaded area*). From *Audiology: Science to practice*, 2nd ed. (Page 259, Figure 8–22) by S. Kramer, 2014, San Diego, CA: Plural Publishing, Inc. Reprinted with permission.

intense or weak OAE at certain frequencies, a concept referred to as fine structure. It is, therefore, important that audiologists interpret OAE cautiously and in the context of other tests and patient history.

TEOAE EVALUATION

- The probe directs the transient stimuli into the ear canal. A microphone transduces OAEs for computer analysis.
- The resulting TEOAE includes intermodulation distortion, at many frequencies requiring computer analysis by fast Fourier transform is beyond the scope of this text.

Interpretation

- TEOAEs should be present above the noise floor by at least 6 dB.
- A minimum wave reproducibility of 50% Kemp, Ryan, and Bray (1990) to 70% Prieve et al. (1993)
- The equipment uses this criteria to recommend "pass" or "refer"

When TEOAE are "pass" at a given frequency, expect normal hearing sensitivity with thresholds at that frequency of roughly 30 dB or better depending on the degree of OHC dysfunction and the integrity of IHC and/or neurons. When TEOAE are "refer" at a given frequency, expect the precipitating OHC disorder to cause at least mild hearing loss at and near that frequency. Specifically, expect audiometric thresholds of roughly 30 dB or poorer depending on the degree of OHC dysfunction and the integrity of IHC and/or neurons.

An example of TEOAE data for a patient with a high-frequency hearing loss is shown in Table 16–2.

Table 16–2. Example of Transient Evoked Otoacoustic Emissions (TOAE) Data for a Patient with Hearing Loss

Frequency (Hz) Assessed	*Reproducibility in %*	*TEOAE (dB SPL)*	*Noise Floor (dB SPL)*	*TEOAE—Noise Floor (dB SPL)*	*Pass/Refer*
1500	39	–2.1	–4.9	2.8	Refer
2000	34	–2.6	–4.5	1.9	Refer
3000	50	–1.8	–5.0	3.2	Refer
4000	27	–3.3	–5.9	2.6	Refer

Figure 16–2 shows an example of patient data plotted on a graph.

Caveat

The first few milliseconds of TEOAE are not analyzed in order to allow the energy from the click

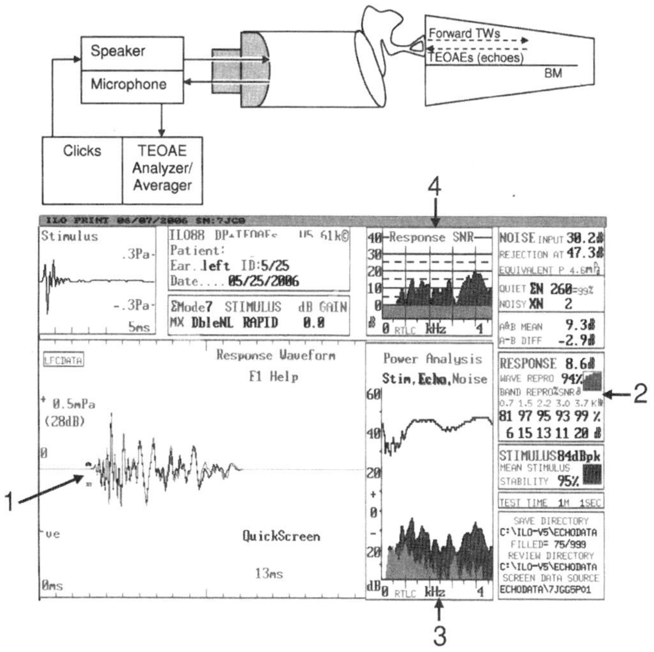

Figure 16–2. *Top:* Diagram of TEOAE apparatus showing a speaker for clicks and a microphone to allow for analysis. *Bottom:* Example data showing (1) TEOAE sound wave with replication, (2) correlation between the two TEOAE, (3) absolute TEOAE amplitude (*dark shading*) rising above noise amplitude (*lighter shading*), (4) TEOAE amplitude (*dark shading*) and noise (*lighter shading*) relative amplitudes. From *Audiology: Science to practice*, 2nd ed. (Page 257, Figure 8–21), by S. Kramer, 2014, San Diego, CA: Plural Publishing, Inc. Reprinted with permission.

to attenuate sufficiently so as not to interfere with TEAOE measurement. This precludes measurement of high frequency emissions from the base of the cochlea, which reach the ear canal within the first few milliseconds. DPOAE is therefore the test of choice for assessing hearing loss at 4000 Hz and higher (Arnold, Lonsbury-Martin & Martin, 1999; Harris & Probst, 1997).

FINAL WORDS

As part of a diagnostic battery, OAE evaluation allows audiologists to diagnose OHC disorder at somewhat specific frequencies. Other tests in the battery must first be used to rule outer and middle ear disorder that precludes OAE evaluation. Still, other tests must be used to assess IHC and/or neural disorder. As a screening tool, OAE evaluation is sensitive to occlusion of the outer ear or middle ear or OHC disorder. OAE alone is not sufficient to differentially diagnose site of lesion.

REFERENCES

Arnold, D. J., Lonsbury-Martin, B. L., & Martin, G. K. (1999). High-frequency hearing influences lower-frequency distortion-product otoacoustic emissions. *Archives of Otolaryngol Head Neck Surgery, 125*(2), 215–222. http://dx.doi.org/10.1001/archotol.125.2.215

Hall, J. W. (2000). *Handbook of otoacoustic emissions*. San Diego, CA: Singular.

Hall, J. W., & Mueller, H. G. (1997). *Audiologists' desk reference*. San Diego, CA: Singular.

Harris F.P., & Probst R. (1997). Otoacoustic emissions and audiometric outcomes. In M. S. Robinette & T. J. Glattke (Eds.), *Otoacoustic emission: Clinical application* (pp. 213–242). New York, NY: Thieme.

Kemp, D. T. (2003). *The OAE story*. (pp. 30–38). Hatfield, Herts, UK: Otodynamics.

Kemp, D. T., Ryan, S., & Bray, P. (1990). A guide to the effective use of otoacoustic emissions. *Ear and Hearing*, *11*(2), 93–105.

Prieve, B. A., Gorga, M. P., Schmidt, A., Neely, S., Peters, J., Schultes, L., & Jesteadt, W. (1993). Analysis of transient-evoked otoacoustic emissions in normal-hearing and hearing-impaired ears. *Journal of the Acoustical Society of America*, *93*(6). http://dx.doi.org/10.1121/1.405715

Withnell, R. H. & Yates G. K. (1998). Enhancement of the transient-evoked otoacoustic emission produced by the addition of a pure-tone in the guinea pig. *Journal of the Acoustical Society of America*, *104*, 344–349.

17

Auditory Evoked Potentials

OVERVIEW

Evoked potentials are electrical signals generated by the nervous system in response to a stimulus, and are used to diagnose a variety of neurological disorders. Auditory evoked potentials (AEPs) are used to evaluate the integrity of the auditory system and to make estimates of hearing sensitivity. A comprehensive discussion of AEPs is beyond the scope of this book. This chapter will focus on the two most common applications of AEPs used in clinical practice, Auditory Brainstem Response (ABR) and Electrocochleography (ECochG.)

The AEPs are generated in response to an acoustic stimulus (click, tone burst, tone pip or chirp) and are typically measured using electrodes on the surface of the skin or on the eardrum. Clicks cause synchronous neural firings evoked from the 1000- to 4000-Hz place in the cochlea. Tone bursts, tone pips or chirp stimuli are more frequency-specific. Trans-tympanic electrodes may also be used in testing such as electrocochleography (EcochG.)

AUDITORY BRAINSTEM RESPONSE (ABR) OR BRAINSTEM AUDITORY EVOKED RESPONSE (BAER)

ABR testing is an objective test that evaluates the integrity of the hearing system from the level of the cochlea ascending through the lower brainstem. First described by Jewitt and Williston (1971), ABR is considered an early onset response potential as it occurs within 10 ms after the onset of the stimulus (Figure 17–1).

ABR is a far-field recorded potential; electrodes are placed on the scalp, mastoid, ear lobe or in the ear canal, far from the potential generator of the response. Recordings typically require three or four electrodes used in an electrode montage. Electrodes are assigned as active (+), reference (–), and ground. The response is recorded from a pair of electrodes, typically Cz or Fz (vertex or high forehead) to A1 (left ear lobe) or A2 (right earlobe).

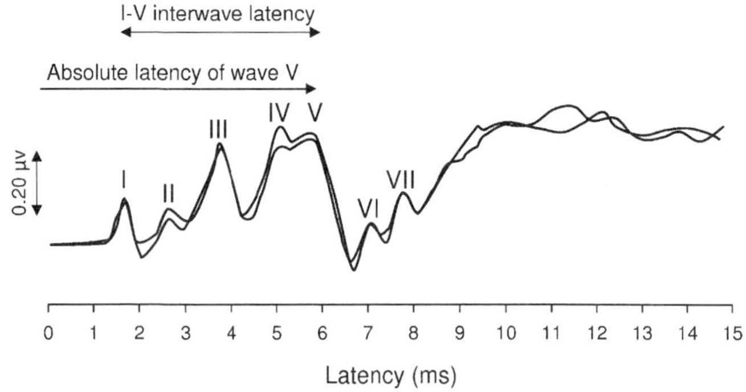

Figure 17–1. Normal latency waves, waves I through VII identified. From *Audiology: Science to practice,* 2nd ed. (Page 261, Figure 8–23), by S. Kramer, 2014, San Diego, CA: Plural Publishing, Inc. Reprinted with permission.

The vertex is the preferred electrode placement site because larger waveform amplitudes can be observed; however, a high forehead or Fz placement is often utilized clinically to avoid interfering with the patient's hair.

To produce a response, the voltages at each of the electrodes are subtracted from each other by the equipment amplifier. Electrical activity (noise) common to both electrodes is cancelled out and only the response voltage remains. This is called common mode rejection. The response voltage is then amplified. It is imperative that low and equal impedance at the electrode sites is obtained for common mode rejection to work well.

PREPARATION FOR TESTING

Room Preparation

In order to avoid electrical interference or noise in the response, several precautions should be taken.

- It is best to utilize a designated and grounded electrical outlet for the evoked potential (EP) equipment.
- EP equipment includes a pre-amplifier. The pre-amp should not be placed near the computer monitor or the isolation transformer/power source for the EP unit.
- Turn off all other computer monitors in the test room.
- If an electrically operated chair is used for height or recline, unplug the chair after it has been adjusted.

- Cell phones should be turned off (not on silent); particularly smartphones that transmit data.
- Turn off or dim fluorescent lights; when necessary use incandescent lighting.

Patient Preparation

- Patient's skin must be exfoliated to prepare for electrode placement.
  - Gels or electrode prep pads, which include fine pumice granules, are used to exfoliate the skin. Gels can be applied with cotton pads or cotton tip applicators.
- After the skin has been prepared, electrode paste or gel is applied to non-disposable cup electrodes before securing to the skin with medical tape. If using disposable electrodes, ensure the skin is dry before applying the electrode.
- Electrodes act like antennas. When separated, each electrode acts like a separate antenna and therefore recordings will be noisier. Braiding the electrodes (or taping them together) will reduce noise.
- Electrode leads should run toward the top of the head for patient comfort and to avoid accidental displacement.
- Avoid electrode leads and transducer cables from crossing. This will reduce artifact in the recording.
- Patients must be quiet during testing; it's best when they are asleep.

Electrode Impedance Measurement

Before beginning the test, electrode impedances must be checked to ensure they are low and balanced. This is critical for common mode rejection to work well. We recommend impedances below 5 kOhms and values between electrodes are within 2 kOhms.

ADULT NEUROLOGICAL ASSESSMENT

Equipment and test parameters (recommendations from Hall, 2007; Hall & Mueller, 1997)

- Transducer: Inserts preferred; supra-aural phones may be used
- Type of stimulus: Click
- Polarity: Rarefaction preferred because it often results in a clear wave I
- Rate: 21.1/sec preferred; slower rate may be used to enhance wave I
- Intensity: Varies based on the 1000 Hz, 2000 Hz, 4000 Hz PTA:
  - 10 to 19 dB PTA = 70 dB nHL
  - 20 to 39 dB PTA = 80 dB nHL
  - 40 to 59 dB PTA = 90 dB nHL
  - 60 to 79 dB PTA = 100 dB nHL, though we recommend caution with intensity levels this high.
- Masking: Necessary when the stimulus is > 70 dB and ABR shows no wave I and delayed wave V latency
- Presentation: Monaural
- Ramping: Blackman
- Epoch: 15 ms
- Filter: 30 to 3000 Hz

- Notch filter: none
- Sample points: 512
- Sweeps: 2000 preferred first run; second run may be stopped if waveform reproducible after 500 sweeps

INFANT HEARING THRESHOLD ESTIMATION

- Transducer: Inserts preferred; supra-aural phones or B-70 bone oscillator may be used
- Type of Stimulus: Click, tone burst, or chirp
- Duration of Stimulus: Click 0.1 ms; tone bursts two cycles of rise and fall
- Polarity: Rarefaction and condensation
- Rate: 21.1/sec preferred; slower rate may be used to enhance wave I
- Intensity: 95 dB nHL down to 0 dB nHL; decrease intensity in 10 to 20 dB steps until no repeatable wave V is seen. ABR threshold is the lowest intensity that wave V is judged to be present (Figure 17–2). For clinical ramifications see Threshold estimation under Basic ABR Interpretation below.
- Masking: Necessary when the stimulus is >70 dB and ABR shows no wave I and delayed wave V latency
- Presentation: Monaural
- Ramping: Blackman
- Epoch: 20 msec
- Filter: 30 to 100 Hz high-pass setting; 2000 to 3000 Hz low-pass setting
- Notch filter: none

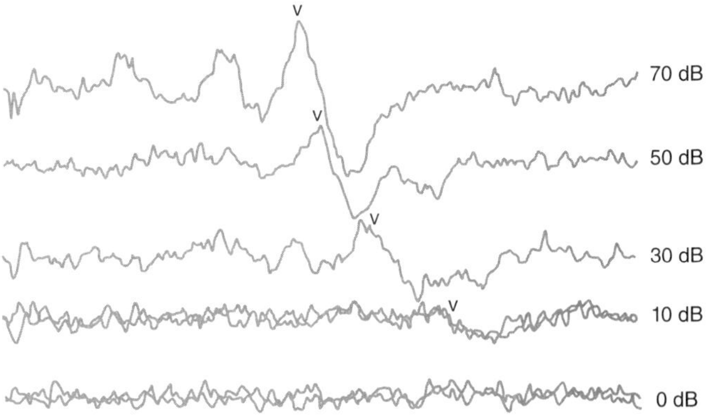

Figure 17–2. The prediction of hearing sensitivity with ABR, showing the tracking of wave V as click intensity level is reduced. From *Clinical audiology: An introduction,* 2nd ed. (Page 372, Figure 9–7), by B. Stach, 2016, San Diego, CA: Plural Publishing, Inc. Reprinted with permission.

- Sample points: 512
- Sweeps: 2000 preferred first run; second run may be stopped if reproducible. Additional sweeps may be necessary closer to patient threshold

SUBJECT FACTORS

Several subject factors must be considered prior to analysis of the response. ABR is incomplete at birth due to several factors including incomplete myelination, reduced axon diameter and immature synaptic functioning. Later waves are affected most. At 18 months to two years ABR response becomes adult-like. As we age and lose neural synapses, the waveform may be adversely affected. In general, females have earlier shorter wave latencies and larger amplitudes than males. This is most noticeable in the later waves.

The subject's state, whether awake or asleep, does not interfere with testing or interpretation. Muscle activity in the jaw and neck area can cause artifact/interference in the recording. This should not be a problem with a relaxed or sleeping patient.

ANALYSIS OF RESPONSE

You will analyze the response to identify the Jewitt/Williston wave I–V sequence. The most common ABR characteristics used to distinguish between normal and abnormal responses are wave component latency (absolute, interwave and interaural wave V latency differences) and amplitude. Differentiation of normal versus abnormal ABR is based on latency of the major waves (I, III, and V). Normative data should be collected for each piece of equipment.

- General rules for absolute latencies are: wave I, 1.5 msec; wave III, 3.5 msec; and wave V, 5.5 msec.
- The interwave latencies should be 2 msec between waves I–III and III–V, and 4 msec between wave 1–V.
- The V/I amplitude ratio must be at least >0.5, ideally >1.0.

Jewitt and Williston (1971) described the neural generator sites for the waves found when recording ABR. While multiple generators are likely involved, the following are generally accepted.

- Wave I: distal portion of the auditory (VIII) nerve, as it emerges from the cochlea
- Wave II: proximal portion of the auditory (VIII) nerve, as it enters the cochlear nucleus
- Wave III: cochlear nucleus
- Wave IV: superior olivary complex
- Wave V: lateral lemniscus
- Waves VI & VII: inferior colliculus

Basic ABR Interpretation (Hall, 2007)

- Normal: Absolute latencies WNL; interpeak latencies WNL; interaural comparison is good
- Threshold estimation: Threshold is 10 to 15 dB below the lowest dB nHL level at which a repeatable wave V is seen.
- Conductive hearing loss: Wave I delayed, all other waves shift accordingly and are also delayed; interpeak latencies WNL; latency-intensity shifts to higher levels by the magnitude of the conductive loss; waveform will look normal at higher intensity levels.
- Severe sensory/cochlear hearing loss: No response at lower stimulus levels; wave I may be absent; abnormally long wave V latencies that get shorter as we reach the highest intensity levels.
- Mild cochlear hearing loss: slightly increased wave I latency with an equivalent increase in later wave components.
- Retrocochlear hearing loss: increased wave I–III suggests the presence of a lesion of

the 8th CN or caudal pons; increased III–V latency suggests presence of a lesion of the rostral pons or midbrain; absence of wave components beyond wave I strongly indicates the presence of retrocochlear pathology; may also have prolongation of absolute and/or interwave latencies; degradation of the waveform, poor waveform reproducibility; absent waveforms; prolonged waves I–V interwave latency.

ELECTROCOCHLEOGRAPHY

Electrocochleography (ECochG) is a method for recording electrical potentials of the cochlea and auditory nerve. The potentials most often recorded in ECochG are the cochlear microphonic (CM), the summating potential (SP), and the action potential (AP) (Figure 17–3). The CM is predominantly generated by the outer hair cells of the organ of Corti. It is an alternating current (AC) voltage that mirrors the waveform of the acoustic stimulus at low-to-moderate levels of stimulation. The SP is a direct current that reflects the time-displacement pattern of the cochlear partition in response to the stimulus envelope (Dallos, 1973). It is also generated primarily by the outer hair cells of the organ of Corti. The AP is an AC potential that represents the summed response of the synchronous firing of several thousand auditory nerve fibers. The response is dominated by high-frequency nerve fibers when generated in response to transient stimuli of rapid onset, like a broadband click. The resulting waves, unlike ABR, are plotted downward (see Figure 17–3). The most popular application of the AP is the measurement

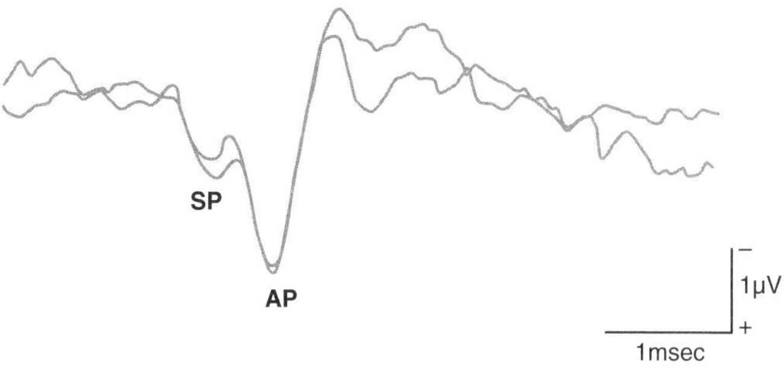

Figure 17–3. ECochG yielding normal summating potential (SP) and action potential (AP). From *Clinical audiology: An introduction,* 2nd ed. (Page 365, Figure 9–4), by B. Stach, 2016, San Diego, CA: Plural Publishing, Inc. Reprinted with permission.

of the magnitude of the response in comparison to the SP in patients suspected of having Meniere's disease or endolymphatic hydrops. Other clinical applications of the ECochG include enhancement of wave I of ABR in the presence of hearing loss, or when wave I could not be recorded in ABR and measurement and monitoring of cochlear and auditory nerve function during surgery involving the auditory periphery.

Preparation for the test, the patient and electrode impedance measurement is similar to what was described earlier in this chapter for ABR. In order to obtain the best response, electrode placement should be as close to the cochlea as possible. Unlike ABR, the ECochG is a near-field response. This means the response is recorded best when an electrode is within the electrode field producing the response. A transtympanic electrode can be placed by an otolaryngologist through the posterior inferior quadrant of the tympanic membrane (TM) to the cochlear promontory. When an audiologist is working independently, a TM electrode is the best choice. A tiptrode, an electrode that sits in the ear canal, may also be used; however, the response is often small and difficult to distinguish due to the proximity to the cochlea. If this is the audiologist's only choice, ensure that the tiptrode is inserted as far into the ear canal as possible.

Equipment and Test Parameters (Hall & Mueller, 1997)

- Transducer: Inserts
- Type of stimulus: Click
- Polarity: Alternating (minimizes the CM)
- Rate: 7.1/sec and 99.9/sec—slow rate for enhanced AP, fast rate to differentiate SP from AP
- Intensity: 90 to 95 dB HL
- Masking: None
- Epoch: 5 to 10 ms
- Filter: 5 or 10 to 1500 Hz
- Notch filter: none
- Sweeps: 500 to 1500 for tiptrode or TM electrodes; 100 to 200 for transtympanic electrode
- Runs: Three or four to verify repeatability
- The amplification factor is 75,000 for tiptrode and TM electrodes; less for transtympanic electrodes

Basic ECochG Interpretation (Ferraro, 2000; Hall & Mueller, 1997)

Assessment of Meniere's disease/endolymphatic hydrops is done through the measurement of the SP and AP. The SP/AP amplitude ratio is derived from the absolute SP and AP amplitudes. Ratios in excess of 0.35 are considered to be abnormal when using a tympanic membrane electrode; >0.50 for tiptrode and >0.30 for transtympanic electrode placements. You must also assess interaural asymmetry in SP/AP ratio and report differences of >10%. While the reported incidence of enlarged SP/AP amplitude ratios in the general Meniere's population is only 60% to 65%, the best way to improve sensitivity of the test is to evaluate the patient when he or she is symptomatic.

For patients with hearing loss, including those with acoustic neuroma's, wave I of ABR may be reduced or absent despite wave V being present. This reduces the clinical utility of ABR as a diagnostic tool. The addition of an ECochG recording in this case may allow comparison of a recorded N1 component with the wave V of ABR recording to assist with determination of site of lesion.

REFERENCES

Dallos P. (1973). *The auditory periphery: Biophysics and physiology*. New York, NY: Academic Press.

Ferraro, J.A. (2000). Clinical electrocochleography: Overview of theories, techniques and applications. *AudiologyOnline,* Article 1275. Retrieved from http//www.audiologyonline.com.

Hall, J. W. (2007). *New handbook of auditory evoked responses*. Upper Saddle River, NJ: Pearson.

Hall, J. W., & Mueller, H. G. (1997). *Audiologists' desk reference: Volume I*. San Diego, CA: Singular.

Jewitt, D., & Williston, J. (1971). Auditory-evoked far fields averaged from the scalp of humans. *Brain, 94*, 681–696.

18

Nonorganic Hearing Loss

OVERVIEW

There are many reasons patients may exhibit nonorganic hearing loss, and a few are discussed below. It is audiologists' responsibility to assess reliability and validity, and in this chapter we cover many of the tests and observations that can be used including:

- Non-test behaviors
- Pure-tone average (PTA)–Speech recognition threshold (SRT) agreement
- Ascending-descending threshold searches
- Audiogram configuration
- Stenger
- Low-level speech and Word recognition score (WRS)
- Yes-no test
- Electrophysiologic tests (auditory brainstem response (ABR), otoacoustic emissions (OAE)

RELIABILITY AND VALIDITY

Many of these observations and tests, especially behavioral tests, involve judgment of response reliability. Reliable results might be valid, but unreliable results cannot be valid. Unreliable results might reflect patient bias fueled by potential gain, for example, adults seeking monetary gain or children seeking attention or an excuse for poor grades. Patient illness, misunderstood directions, or equipment malfunction might also affect reliability and/or validity. Regardless of cause, unreliable results must be identified so as not to lead to an erroneous conclusion that results are valid. The potential ramifications of error include but are not limited to:

- The completion of unnecessary and expensive medical tests or procedures
- The ordering of hearing aids when none are needed
- The unwarranted awarding of workers compensation, veterans affairs service connection, or other benefit
- The unwarranted impact in the education setting, including teacher-parent meetings, classroom modification, and the unnecessary initiation of an individual education plan
- Unnecessarily causing worry among family and friends
- The adverse impact on audiologists' professional standing

TERMS

Recommended terms include nonorganic hearing loss, pseudohypoacusis, and functional hearing loss. Functional and nonorganic suggest hearing loss without an identifiable cause (site-of-lesion). Pseudohypoacusis, sometimes spelled pseudohypacusis, essentially translates to false-poor hearing. Audiologists should avoid terms that imply intent to deceive, including malingering, feigning, and faking. Intent cannot be known or diagnosed by audiologists. Psychological terms such as psychogenic or hysterical hearing loss are reserved for use by mental health providers.

NON-TEST BEHAVIORS

- Be wary of exaggerated struggling-to-hear behaviors.
- Be wary of inconsistencies in the case history. For example, it is unreasonable for a patient with profound hearing loss to have never sought evaluation and to not be using hearing aids.
- Ask questions of the patient without visual cues, for example, when looking away or when switching ears during otoscopy; consider whether their ability to understand the questions is consistent with test results.
- Finally, when possible, observe interactions with office staff and family members and consider whether their ability to communicate is consistent with test results.

BEHAVIORAL TEST RESPONSE RELIABILITY

- Audiometers are calibrated such that the speech recognition threshold (SRT) will agree with the three-frequency pure-tone average (PTA) at 500 Hz, 1000 Hz, and 2000 Hz. Typically agreement within +/−6 dB is considered good agreement and suggest a reliable PTA, 7 to 12 dB fair agreement/reliability, and >13 dB difference poor agreement/reliability. However, this might not hold true when one or two of the PTA thresholds is at least 20 dB poorer an adjacent threshold. In such cases, the SRT should be compared, with caution, to a PTA of the two best PTA thresholds.
- Half-word responses during SRT testing should be viewed with suspicion. Audiologists should accordingly note when patients offer half-word responses, but only accept a response when both syllables are correctly repeated.
- A 1000-Hz air conduction test–retest reliability should be within +/−5 dB.
- Audiologists can abandon traditional "10 down 5 up" threshold search in favor of an ascending threshold search, followed by a descending threshold search at any test frequency. For the ascending run, start at 0 dB and ascend slowly and deliberately, preferably in 2-dB steps or even 1-dB steps. A similarly slow and deliberate descending run should follow, beginning well above the suspected thresholds; the two threshold searches should be separated

by a diversionary pause in order to disrupt patient memory of tone loudness. To be considered reliable, the two threshold searches should yield thresholds within +/−5 dB.

AUDIOGRAM CONFIGURATION

- Etiology specific audiogram patterns: Patients with nonorganic hearing loss do not understand that for a given etiology, certain audiogram patterns are expected, whereas others are not. For example, patients with noise-induced hearing loss typically present with a 3000 Hz-, 4000 Hz-, or 6000 Hz-notched audiogram rather than a flat or rising audiogram. Instead, a patient with nonorganic hearing loss might respond similarly to tones at all frequencies, thus yielding a flat audiogram pattern.
- Shadow audiogram pattern: High-intensity tones presented to one ear should cross over and be heard in the other ear (see Chapter 4). In patients with unilateral hearing loss, the resulting audiogram pattern will, therefore, show poorer ear thresholds mirroring better ear thresholds by the amount of interaural attenuation, a so-called "shadow audiogram." In a patient with unilateral, *nonorganic* hearing loss, a shadow audiogram will not be seen. This is because high-intensity tones presented to the "poorer" ear are louder than admitted

to, and crossover is not perceived due to the Stenger effect (see below). Audiologists should be suspicious when there is no evidence of crossover. The astute audiologist will understand that supra aural earphones are the earphone of choice because of their low interaural attenuation.

STENGER

The Stenger test is used for unilateral or asymmetric hearing loss of at least 20 dB, though we find 30 or even 40 dB asymmetry is more amenable. The pure-tone Stenger test relies on the Stenger principle: When two tones of the same frequency are introduced simultaneously to both ears, only the louder tone will be perceived (Martin & Clark, 2015).

Pure-Tone Stenger Screening

- Present a tone simultaneously 10 dB above the better ear threshold (10 dB SL) and 10 dB below the poorer ear threshold. The patient with a true unilateral hearing loss will hear the tone in the better ear and respond. The tone in the poorer ear is not audible. In contrast, if the patient is feigning unilateral hearing loss, the tone in the "poorer" ear is audible and it dominates patient's perception (the Stenger principle). But because he or she does not want to admit to hearing the tone in that "poorer" ear he or she does not respond.

Stenger Threshold Estimation Using the Minimum Interference Level

- Present tones simultaneously to each ear, one at 10 dB SL in the "better" ear, and another at 0 dB HL in the "poorer" ear. The patient will respond to the tone heard in the "better" ear.
- Continue with simultaneous tone presentations, maintaining the 10 dB SL tone in the "better" ear but raising the tone in the poorer ear in 5-dB increments.
- When the tone in the "poorer" ear is loud enough to evoke the Stenger principle, the nonorganic patient will stop responding so as not to give away the fact the he or she heard the tone in that ear. This "minimum contralateral interference level" (MCIL) is typically 15 to 20 dB above true threshold in the "poorer" ear.

Speech Stenger

Stenger screening and MCIL testing can be conducted with spondees in a manner similar to that described for tones.

LOW-LEVEL WRS

Nonorganic hear loss patients might have a difficult time judging word intensity, and may therefore show better than expected word recognition at intensities near their SRT, or even (rarely) below their SRT.

Better-than-expected word recognition within 10 or 20 dB of SRT is suspicious.

YES-NO TEST

Children can sometimes be instructed by the audiologist to "say yes when you hear the tone and say no when you don't." Thus a "no" response is an indication a tone was heard. An audiogram can thus be completed on a child who believes he or she is not cooperating.

ELECTROPHYSIOLOGIC TESTS

Electrophysiologic tests are objective measures, some of which can be used to estimate hearing sensitivity. Electrophysiologic tests are generally excellent for extreme cases for example, patients with normal hearing who are feigning at least moderate hearing loss. However, electrophysiologic tests are generally not sensitive to smaller exaggerations of hearing loss. Also, electrophysiologic tests require hearing; patients with severe to profound hearing loss might not have enough usable hearing for electrophysiologic tests to be an option.

Some of the electrophysiologic tests available are listed below, though procedures and interpretation are covered in other chapters.

- Acoustic reflex thresholds
- Broadband noise acoustic reflex threshold screening
- Sensitivity prediction by acoustic reflexes
- 10th percentile acoustic reflex norms

- Acoustic reflex thresholds below admitted hearing thresholds
- Otoacoustic emissions
- Auditory brainstem response and other evoked potentials

REFERENCE

Martin, F. N., & Clark, J. G. (2015). Nonorganic hearing loss. In J. Katz (Ed.), *Handbook of clinical audiology* (7th ed., pp. 617–630). Philadelphia, PA: Wolters Kluwer.

19

Tinnitus Evaluation

OVERVIEW

Patients with the primary complaint of tinnitus may benefit from a tinnitus evaluation for at least four reasons.

1. First, a thorough evaluation will show the patient your intent to address his or her complaints directly, while assuring him or her you have the test data to do so effectively.
2. Second, audiologists armed with data from a tinnitus evaluation may be better positioned to choose the sound therapy to mask or partially mask the tinnitus.
3. Third, data from a tinnitus evaluation might help audiologists determine prognosis. Prognosis might be best when the tinnitus is amenable to sound therapy.
4. Fourth, hyperacusis often accompanies tinnitus, and hyperacusis measurement is often a part of a tinnitus evaluation. Hyperacusis can cause patients to reject sound therapy, so its identification and treatment are essential.

CASE HISTORY AND TINNITUS HANDICAP INVENTORY (THI)

A case history will allow audiologists to obtain important information on the subjective tinnitus cause, laterality, pitch, and loudness. Audiologists can also ascertain exacerbating or mitigating factors, perceived handicap, and readiness for treatment. Many tools are available to help audiologists obtain some of this information; we recommend the THI (Newman, Sandridge, & Jacobson, 1998). The THI is a standardized tool for assessing handicap and monitoring the effect of treatment. It is a paper and pencil assessment tool that categorizes tinnitus severity. The THI reliability is documented, and it can be used as a standardized assessment of measured outcomes.

THI Scoring

THI scoring: 25 questions, 100 points:

- Severe tinnitus = 58 to 100
- Moderate tinnitus = 38 to 56
- Mild tinnitus = 18 to 36
- No tinnitus handicap >18
- Post treatment re-test: >20-point change is significant

THI screening can be used to save time. THI screening scoring: 10 items, 40 points:

- Score of >6 suggests need for tinnitus management

- Post treatment re-test: >10-point change is significant

LOUDNESS DISCOMFORT LEVEL

Loudness discomfort level assessment can help the audiologist identify hyperacusis, and identify appropriate output limiting settings on treatment devices such as hearing aids and noise generators.

Procedure

There are several procedures for measuring loudness discomfort. We recommend a procedure adapted from Henry, Zaugg, and Schechter (2005).

- Test each ear separately, at 1000 Hz, 2000 Hz, 4000 Hz, and 8000 Hz
- Begin at approximate MCL or 20 dB below expected LDL and deliver 1- to 2-second tones in 5-dB ascending steps
- Loudness discomfort: Patient indicates when tones cannot be tolerated for more than 3 seconds; this is the loudness discomfort level.

TINNITUS LOUDNESS MATCHING AND PITCH MATCHING

Tinnitus loudness matching can be used by the audiologist in the determination of prognosis; softer tinnitus is more easily masked or partially masked as desired. Moreover, masking and partial masking is more likely when the tinnitus pitch is within the frequency output range of sound therapy devices.

Loudness and Pitch Matching Procedure

Adapted from Henry, Zaugg, and Schechter (2005).

- Start: Identify a tinnitus and stimuli ear. The tinnitus ear has the loudest tinnitus; if equal, choose arbitrarily. Present tones to the opposite ear, called the stimuli ear.
- Tinnitus pitch match: Communicate with patient while changing frequency to determine pitch match. Final check: Patient pitch matches can be off by one octave; compare the measured pitch match to a tone one octave higher to ensure pitch match accuracy.
- Tinnitus quality match: Compare narrow band noise and tone at pitch match frequency to determine which stimuli better matches the tinnitus.
- Tinnitus loudness match: At the pitch match frequency, and using the best match of tone or narrow band noise, communicate with patient while adjusting intensity in 1-dB steps until tinnitus loudness is matched.

TINNITUS MINIMUM MASKING LEVEL

Tinnitus minimum masking level (MML) is a measure of whether tinnitus can be masked or partially masked, and therefore inform treatment prognosis.

MML Procedure

Adapted from Henry, Zaugg, and Schechter (2005).

- Present white noise binaurally if tinnitus is binaural, present white noise unilaterally in the tinnitus ear if tinnitus is unilateral. Measure a white-noise threshold in 1-dB ascending steps.
- MML: Beginning at white-noise threshold, and raise white noise in 1-dB steps until tinnitus is masked; document the MML in dB SL and dB HL.
- If tinnitus is masked in one ear only, raise the white noise in the other ear only and in 1-dB steps until the tinnitus is masked. Document the MML in dB SL and dB HL.

RESIDUAL INHIBITION

Residual inhibition (RI) is a sustained diminishing of tinnitus loudness after withdrawal of masking. Patients who exhibit residual inhibition might have a better prognosis for benefit from sound therapy than do patients without residual inhibition or with less residual inhibition.

RI Procedure

Adapted from Henry, Zaugg, and Schechter (2005).

- Present white noise at MML + 10 dB for one minute. Immediately communicate with patient to determine if tinnitus has changed.

- RI: Document as complete residual inhibition (tinnitus is not heard), partial residual inhibition (tinnitus loudness is reduced), or no residual inhibition.
- RI time: Communicate with patient to determine when tinnitus has returned to normal loudness from 0 to 4 minutes (there is no need to document longer RI times).

REFERENCES

Henry, J. A., Zaugg, T. L., & Schechter, M. A. (2005). Clinical guide for audiologic tinnitus management I: Assessment. *American Journal of Audiology*, *14*, 21–48.

Newman, C. W., Jacobson, G. P., & Spitzer, J. B. (1996). Development of the Tinnitus Handicap Inventory. *Archives of Otolaryngology Head and Neck Surgery 122*, 143–148.

Newman, C. W., Sandridge, & S. A., Jacobson, G.P. (1998). Psychometric adequacy of the Tinnitus Handicap Inventory (THI) for evaluating treatment outcome. *Journal of the American Academy of Audiology*, *9*, 153–160.

20

(Central) Auditory Processing

OVERVIEW

(Central) auditory processing (C)AP refers to the efficiency and effectiveness of the central nervous system (CNS) to utilize auditory information. The American Speech-Language Hearing Association (ASHA, 2005) Working Group on Auditory Processing Disorders defined a (C)APD

> *. . . as difficulties in the perceptual processing of auditory information in the CNS as demonstrated by poor performance in one or more of the following auditory skills: sound localization and lateralization; auditory discrimination; auditory pattern recognition; temporal aspects of audition, including temporal integration, temporal discrimination (e.g., temporal gap detection), temporal ordering, and temporal masking; auditory performance in competing acoustic signals (including dichotic listening); and auditory performance with degraded acoustic signals.*

Although other auditory skills (i.e., auditory synthesis, phonological awareness, etc.) may be dependent on central auditory processing ability, they are considered to be higher order cognitive-communicative and/or language related functions and are not included in the definition of (C)AP.

A diagnosis of (C)APD should only result when a deficit in the central auditory nervous system (CANS) can be demonstrated. The differential diagnosis can be difficult as basic neuroscience indicates there are few, if any, compartmentalized areas in the brain solely responsible for a single sensory modality (Poremba et al., 2003; Salvi et al., 2002). A test battery approach, in addition to a thorough case history, will provide the necessary information to identify the presence of abnormalities in the CANS and to describe the extent of the disorder. Test results will also help guide the appropriate management and intervention programs for the patient.

CASE HISTORY

(C)APD have been associated with a number of neurological lesions and degenerative diseases, such as multiple sclerosis, seizure disorders, and head trauma. Additionally, neuromaturational delays in the development of the CANS, secondary to auditory deprivation, and age-related changes may cause a CANS dysfunction. A thorough case history can help identify potential etiologies, and the impact the disorder has on the patient's vocational, academic, and communicative function. In addition to the case history, direct observation of the patient's behaviors during the case history, reports from teachers, parents, family members or employers will provide additional insight regarding the patient's deficits. A number of self-assessment tools and behavioral checklists are available and can be helpful in providing a systematic review of potential behaviors or symptoms consistent with (C)APD.

PATIENT CRITERIA

- Age: 7 years of age or older (a limited number of behavioral measures have been developed for younger children)
- Cognitive abilities: Normal cognitive status (for patients with impaired cognition, modifying test procedures may be possible for the skilled clinician)
- Medications: If medications have been prescribed for attention, anxiety, of other cognitive disorders, patient should remain on medications for most evaluations unless evaluating the effectiveness of medications is the goal of the evaluation.
- Language Status: Native English speaker; non-native speakers may require modifications to the test battery.
- Speech Intelligibility: Adequate speech production skills are required to interpret results accurately.
- Peripheral Hearing Loss: Normal hearing is required on many tests, 20 to 25 dB HL thresholds or better; mild to moderate hearing loss with good speech recognition abilities may be candidates for some select tests within the (C)APD battery.

SCREENING ASSESSMENTS

Both children and adults suspected of having (C)APD should be screened. Although additional screening tools are needed, it is our recommendation that subtests of the SCAN-3A and SCAN-3C, as well as dichotic digits and speech-in-noise tests, may help identify individuals who should be referred for diagnostic evaluation.

BEHAVIORAL TESTS

Behavioral test batteries used to diagnose (C)APD should include speech and non-verbal tasks in order to evaluate the auditory processes described in the ASHA (2005) definition. Audiologists should choose at least one from each of the following sections in Table 20–1.

Auditory discrimination tests are also recommended as part of the (C)APD test battery. There are no commercially available tests designed for use by audiologists. Speech-language pathologists may have auditory discrimination tests that are part of their test battery.

Table 20–1. Tests of Auditory Processing

Selected Tests of Temporal Processing			
Test	***Process(es) Assessed***	***Sensitive to***	***Source***
Gaps-in-Noise (GIN)	Temporal Resolution	Cortical and brainstem lesions	Musiek et al. (2005)
Random Gap Detection (RGDT)	Temporal Resolution	Cortical lesions, particularly left temporal lobe lesions	Keith (2000)
Frequency Pattern Test (FPT)	Frequency Discrimination, Temporal Ordering, Linguistic Labeling	Cortical lesions, interhemispheric transfer	Musiek (1994)
Duration Pattern Test (DPT)	Duration Discrimination, Temporal Ordering, Linguistic Labeling	Cortical lesions, interhemispheric transfer	Musiek (1994)
Psychoacoustic Pattern Discrimination Test	Temporal Discrimination	Cortical lesions, including auditory association areas	Blaettner, Scherg, & von Cramon (1989)

continues

Table 20–1. *continued*

Selected Dichotic Tests			
Test	***Process(es) Assessed***	***Sensitive to***	***Source***
Dichotic Digits (DD)	Binaural Integration	Brainstem, cortical, and corpus callosal lesions	Musiek (1983)
Dichotic Consonant-Vowels (DC-V)	Binaural Integration	Cortical lesions	Hynd Cohen, & Obrzut (1983)
Staggered Spondaic Word Test (SSW)	Binaural Integration	Brainstem and cortical lesions	Katz, Basil, & Smith (1963)
Competing Sentences (as part of SCAN-3: C or A)	Binaural Separation	Neuromaturation and language processing	Keith (2009)
Synthetic Sentence Identification Test with Contralateral Competing Messages (SSI-CCM)	Binaural Separation	Cortical versus brainstem lesions	Jerger & Jerger (1974)
Dichotic Sentence Identification Test	Binaural Integration	Brainstem and cortical lesions	Noffsinger, Wilson, & Musiek (1994)
Dichotic Rhyme Test	Binaural Integration	Interhemispheric transfer	Musiek et al. (1989)

Selected Monaural Low-Redundancy Speech Tests

Test	***Process(es) Assessed***	***Sensitive to***	***Source***
Low-Pass Filtered Speech (as part of SCAN-3: C or A)	Auditory Closure	Brainstem and cortical lesions, especially primary auditory cortex	Keith (2009)
Time-Compressed Speech (as part of SCAN-3: C or A)	Auditory Closure	Brainstem and cortical lesions, primary auditory cortex	Keith (2009)
Synthetic Sentence Identification Test with Ipsilateral Competing Messages (SSI-ICM)	Auditory Figure Ground, Auditory Closure	Low brainstem lesions	Jerger & Jerger (1974)
Speech-in-Noise (as part of SCAN-3: C or A)	Auditory Figure Ground, Auditory Closure	Low brainstem and cortical issues	Keith (2009)

continues

Table 20–1. *continued*

Selected Tests of Localizations and Lateralization and Other Binaural (Interaction) Tests			
Test	***Process(es) Assessed***	***Sensitive to***	***Source***
Rapidly Alternating Speech Perception (RASP)	Binaural Interaction	Questionable sensitivity to gross brainstem lesions	Willeford (1976)
Binaural Fusion	Binaural Interaction	Gross sensitivity to brainstem lesions	Musiek et al. (1989)
Masking Level Difference (MLD)	Binaural Interaction	Lower brainstem function	Hirsch (1948)
Listening in Spatialized Noise-Sentences Test (LISN-N)	Spatial Aspects of Audition	Lower brainstem function	Cameron, Dillon, & Newall (2006)

ELECTROPHYSIOLOGIC MEASURES

Auditory Brainstem Response (ABR), as previously described in Chapter 17 of this book, is an evoked potential that may be used to provide additional information about the integrity of the auditory nerve and brainstem pathways. One advantage in including ABR in the (C)APD test battery is that ABR has a well-documented maturational response that can be seen at 18 months of age; however, the value of the test remains limited in the diagnosis of (C)APD. Other middle latency and cortical evoked response testing shows promise, especially for younger children who cannot be assessed with traditional behavioral testing. Auditory evoked response testing is not routinely applied in the diagnosis of (C)APD and further research is needed.

INTERPRETATION OF RESULTS

Normative data is provided with test materials for the behavioral tests described above. Additional normative data can be accessed in other texts dedicated to the topic of auditory processing disorders. Most audiology experts in clinical assessment of (C)APD agree that a score of two standard deviations below the mean for at least one ear on at least two different behavioral central auditory tests would support the diagnosis of a (C)APD. In addition to using normative cutoff scores, ear advantage scores can be strong indicators of hemispheric dominance for language, and may suggest neurologically based language/learning disorders (e.g., Keith, 1983). Children with typically developing auditory systems will often exhibit similar right- and left-ear scores on tests of degraded signals, but will have a right-ear advantage on dichotic speech tests. This right-ear advantage diminishes as the child's auditory system matures. Typically, by age 12, the scores are similar in both the right and left ears. When results suggest the continuation of a right- or left-ear advantage, even with cutoff scores within normal limits, this may indicate a (C)APD.

REFERENCES

American Speech-Language-Hearing Association. (2005). *(Central) auditory processing disorders* [Technical report]. Retrieved from http://www.asha.org/docs/html/TR2005-00043.html

Blaettner, U., Scherg, M., & von Cramon, D. (1989) Diagnosis of unilateral telencephalic hearing disorders. Evaluation of a simple psychoacoustic pattern discrimination test. *Brain, 112*(Pt.1), 177–195.

Cameron, S., Dillon, H., & Newall, P. (2006). Development and evaluation of the Listening in Spatialized Noise Test. *Ear and Hearing, 27*, 30–42.

Hirsh, I. J. (1948). Binaural summation and interaural inhibition as a function of the level of the masking noise. *Journal of the Acoustical Society of America, 56*, 205–213.

Hynd. G. W., Cohen. M., & Obrzut, J. E. (1983). Dichotic consonant-vowel (CV) testing in the diagnosis of learning disabilities in children. *Ear and Hearing, 4*, 283–286.

Jerger, J., & Jerger, S. (1974). Auditory findings in brain stem disorders. *Archives of Otolarngology, 99*, 342–350.

Katz, J., Basil, R. A., & Smith, J. M. (1963). A staggered spondaic word test for detecting central auditory lesions. *Annals of Otology, Rhinology & Laryngology, 72*, 908–917.

Keith, R. (1983). Interpretation of the Staggered Spondaic Word test. *Ear and Hearing, 4*(6), 287–292.

Keith, R. (2000). *Random gap detection test.* St. Louis, MO: Auditec.

Keith, R. (2009). *SCAN-3:A tests for auditory processing disorders in adolescents and adults.* San Antonio, TX: Pearson.

Keith, R. (2009). *SCAN-3:C tests for auditory processing disorders for children.* San Antonio, TX: Pearson.

Musiek, F. E. (1983). Assessment of central auditory dysfunction: The dichotic digit test revisited. *Ear and Hearing, 4*, 79–83.

Musiek, F. E. (1994). Frequency (pitch) and duration pattern tests. *Journal of the American Academy of Audiology, 5*, 265–268

Musiek, F. E., Kurdziel-Schwan, S., Kibbe, K. S., Gollegly, K. M., Baran, J. A., & Rintelmann, W. F. (1989). The dichotic rhyme test; results in split-brain patients. *Ear and Hearing, 10*, 33–39.

Musiek, F. E., Shinn, J. B., Jirsa, R., Bamiou, D. E., Baran, J. A., & Zaidan, E. (2005). GIN (Gaps-In-Noise) test performance in subjects with confirmed central auditory nervous system involvement. *Ear and Hearing, 26*, 608–618.

Noffsinger, D., Wilson, R. H., & Musiek, F. E. (1994). Department of Veterans Affairs compact disc recording for auditory perceptual assessment: Background and introduction. *Journal of the American Academy of Audiology, 5*(4), 231–235.

Poremba, A., Saunders, R. C., Crane, A. M., Cook, M., Sokoloff, L., & Mishkin, M. (2003). Functional mapping of the primate auditory system. *Science, 299*, 568–571.

Salvi, R. J., Lockwood, A. H., Frisina, R. D., Coad, M. L., Wack, D. S., & Frisina, D. R. (2002). PET imaging of the normal human auditory system: Responses to speech in quiet and in background noise. *Hearing Research, 170*, 96–106.

Willeford, J. (1976). Differential diagnosis of central auditory dysfunction. In L. Bradford (Ed.), *Audiology: An audio journal for continuing education* (Vol. 2). New York, NY. Grune & Stratton.

21

Middle Ear Disorders

OTITIS MEDIA

Otitis media is typically the result of infection of the eustachian tube and/or middle ear space, although eustachian tube dysfunction can also be caused by allergies and structural abnormalities (Sautter & Hirose, 2007). Otitis media can be divided into at least three general categories: otitis media (a.k.a. eustachian tube dysfunction with or without effusion, serous otitis media), acute otitis media, and chronic otitis media. The audiologist's role is to identify the site of lesion, the likelihood of infection, the need for referral when appropriate, and the need for audiologic monitoring.

When stimulating an ear with otitis media, expect air conduction threshold loss of no more than 60 dB in adults. In contrast, bone conduction thresholds might be normal, resulting in air-bone threshold gaps characteristic of middle ear disorder. However, otitis media might affect bone conduction thresholds to some degree. Yasan (2007) reported 1000 Hz, and in some cases 2000 Hz bone conduction notches analogous to the 2000 Hz Carhart notch seen with ossicular fixation. Similarly, Kumar,

Maheshwar, Mahendran, Oluwasamni, and Clayton (2003) reported 2000 Hz bone conduction notches in patients with viscous effusion. Apparently, effusion can produce stiffening or loading effect in the middle ear, and thus hindering the middle ear bone conduction component (Tonndorf, 1968).

Y226 Hz tympanograms might show some combination of negative pressure, low admittance, and wide widths. The B/G 678 and B/G 1000 Hz tympanograms might be multipeaked >5B and >3G (Harris, Hutchinson, & Moravec, 2005), wide, or even flat. Acoustic reflex thresholds will be elevated by the amount of the air-bone gap when stimulating a disordered ear and absent when measuring in a disordered ear. Otoacoustic emissions (OAE) might be reduced amplitude or absent, depending on the degree of hearing loss, and at frequencies where there is hearing loss. Auditory brainstem response (ABR) waves will be delayed.

Hypothetically, middle ear pathogens can pass through the round window and cause damage to cochlear hair cells, most likely at the basal turn of the cochlea, and thus causing high-frequency sensory/neural hearing loss (Paparella et al., 1984). For an overview of expectations, see Table 21–1.

Table 21–1. Otitis Media

Primary presenting symptom(s)	Gradual onset hearing loss (OME) or onset within 48 hours (AOM) aural fullness or otalgia
Otoscopy	Variable, expect one or more of the following: tympanic membrane retraction, fluid line or bubbles, erythema

Table 21–1. *continued*

Weber tuning fork test	Bone conducted tones might be heard on the affected side in unilateral or asymmetric cases
Pure-tone thresholds	Air-bone gaps, possible bone conduction notch at 1000 Hz or more rarely at 2000 (see Figure 26–1 in Chapter 26)
WRS	Good to excellent
Y226 Hz tympanometry	Expect one or more of the following: negative pressure, low admittance, wide width
B/G 678 and B/G 1000 Hz tympanometry and middle ear resonance	Tympanograms might be multipeaked; >3B and >3G (Wiley, Oviatt, & Block, 1987) >5B and/or >3G is definitely abnormal (Harris, Hutchinson, & Moravec, 2005). Low admittance and wide width are possible. Resonant peak can be high when effusion stiffens the ear or low when effusion viscosity adds mass.
Acoustic reflex thresholds	Acoustic reflex thresholds will be elevated by the amount of the air-bone gap when stimulating a disordered ear and absent when measuring in a disordered ear.
Wideband acoustic immittance (WAI)	Narrow high-frequency reflectance notch at 3000 Hz or above (Feeney, Grant, & Marryott, 2003), flat in cases of excessive effusion
Distortion product otoacoustic emissions (DPOAE)	Reduced amplitude or absent at frequencies where there is hearing loss, depending on the degree of hearing loss
Auditory evoked potentials	Delayed wave latency
Differential diagnosis	Ossicular fixation, ossicular discontinuity, superior semicircular canal dehiscence (SSCD)

OSSICULAR DISCONTINUITY

Ossicular discontinuity is a disorder caused by trauma or, more rarely, chronic middle ear infection. The discontinuity might occur at a middle ear joint or the long process of the malleus or incus. With ossicular discontinuity, the amplifying (impedance matching) role of the middle ear is lost.

When stimulating an ear with ossicular discontinuity, expect air conduction threshold loss up to 60 dB. In contrast, bone conduction thresholds might be normal, resulting in air-bone threshold gaps characteristic of middle ear disorder.

Expect Y226 Hz tympanograms will show high static admittance reflecting middle ear hyperflaccidity. Resonant peak will be lowered by the effect of gravity weighing down the ossicles. Nakajima et al. (2012) reported that ossicular fixation, superior semicircular canal dehiscence (SSCD), and ossicular discontinuity are the only three disorders that manifest as air-bone gaps on the audiogram in patients with normally aerated middle ears (normal middle ear pressure); however, somewhat similar findings have been reported for patients with large vestibular aqueducts (Attias et al., 2012; Merchant, Rosowski, & McKenna, 2007). The B/G 678 and B/G 1000 Hz tympanograms are characteristically multipeaked, the lateral most peaks >75 daPa apart on three-peaked tympanograms and >100 daPa apart on five-peaked tympanograms.

Acoustic reflex thresholds will be elevated by the amount of the air-bone gap when stimulating a disordered ear, and absent when measuring in a disordered ear. OAE will be reduced amplitude or absent, depending on the degree of hearing loss and at frequencies where there is hearing loss. Expect ABR waves to be delayed. For an overview of expectations, see Table 21–2.

Table 21–2. Ossicular Discontinuity

Primary presenting symptom(s)	Onset post physical trauma to the head or chronic ear infection
Otoscopy	Possible co-morbid indicators such as hematotympanum
Weber tuning fork test	Bone conducted tones might be heard on the affected side in unilateral or asymmetric cases
Pure-tone thresholds	Significant air-bone gaps; larger in the 1000–4000 range when compared to SSCD or ossicular fixation (Nakajima, 2012) (see Figure 26–2 in Chapter 26)
WRS	Good to excellent
Y226 Hz tympanometry	High static admittance reflecting hyper-flaccidity
B/G 678 and B/G 1000 Hz tympanometry and middle ear resonance	Expect multi-peaked B/G 678 and B/G 1000 Hz tympanograms (5B5G, 3B5G, or 5B3G), the lateral most peaks >75 daPa apart on 3-peaked tympanograms and >100 daPa apart on 5-peaked tympanograms. Expect low middle ear resonance.
Acoustic reflex thresholds	Acoustic reflex thresholds will be elevated by the amount of the air-bone gap when stimulating a disordered ear and absent when measuring in a disordered ear.
Wideband acoustic immittance (WAI)	Low frequency reflectance notch below 1000 Hz (Feeney, Grant, & Marryott, 2003; Nakajima et al., 2012)
Distortion product otoacoustic emissions (DPOAE)	Reduced amplitude or absent at frequencies where there is hearing loss, depending on the degree of hearing

continues

Table 21–2. *continued*

Auditory evoked potentials	Expect ABR waves to be delayed
Differential diagnosis	Otitis media, ossicular fixation, superior semicircular canal dehiscence (SSCD)

GLOMUS TUMOR

Glomus tumors are benign, slow-growing, highly vascular neoplasms that arise from cells of the paraganglia (Pluta & Iuliano, 2015). For the purposes of this text, only glomus tumors that affect the middle ear space will be discussed; in such cases 80% of patients present with pulsatile tinnitus and 60% present with hearing loss (AAO-HNS, 2014). If cranial nerves become involved, symptoms might include difficulty swallowing, and weakness or paralysis of the face (Pluta & Iuliano, 2015). Glomus tumors of this nature can be divided into two categories: Glomus tympanicum, which develop along the promontory in the middle ear space, and glomus jugulare, which arise from the jugular bulb within the temporal bone and may invade the middle ear space (Silman & Silverman, 1991). The majority of cases of glomus tumors occur in females between the ages of 40 and 60 years (Jerger & Jerger, 1981), and they are present almost exclusively unilaterally.

When the middle ear is affected, testing of air-conduction thresholds could yield hearing loss up to 60 dB, whereas bone conduction thresholds can be normal, resulting in air-bone gaps. In the event that a tumor invades the cochlea, pure-tone threshold results will indicate a mixed hearing loss and thresholds could exceed 60 dB.

Depending on the size and location of a tumor, Y226 Hz tympanograms may show negative pressure, low admittance, wide widths, and normal ear canal volume (Hunter & Sanford, 2015). Acoustic reflex thresholds will be elevated by the amount of the air-bone gap when stimulating a disordered ear and absent when measuring in a disordered ear. Expect OAE to show reduced amplitude or absent, depending on the degree of hearing loss and at frequencies where there is hearing loss. For an overview of expectations, see Table 21–3.

Table 21–3. Glomus Tumor

Primary presenting symptom(s)	Pulsatile tinnitus, hearing loss (AAO-HNS, 2014) vertigo, aural fullness, otalgia, difficulty swallowing, and weakness or paralysis of the face (Pluta & Luliano, 2015)
Otoscopy	Pulsating, red mass behind the TM (glomus tympanicum: Hall & Ghorayeb, 1991) or blue mass behind the TM (glomus jugulare: Northern & English, 1991)
Weber tuning fork test	Bone conducted tones might be heard on the affected side
Pure-tone thresholds	Air-bone gaps (see Figure 26–3), a sensorineural component may be present if tumor has reached the inner ear

continues

Table 21–3. *continued*

WRS	Good to excellent if solely a conductive impairment, can be poorer if a sensorineural component (mixed loss) is present
Y226 Hz tympanometry	Variable depending on size and location of tumor, results can range from within normal limits to negative pressure, low admittance, and wide width
B/G 678 and B/G 1000 Hz tympanometry and middle ear resonance	Tumor might create a mass-dominated middle ear, resonant peak will likely be low and B/G 678 and B/G 1000 Hz tympanometry may indicate multipeaked traces (Hunter & Sanford, 2015) or flat with B greater than G.
Acoustic reflex thresholds	Acoustic reflex thresholds will be elevated by the amount of the air-bone gap when stimulating a disordered ear and absent when measuring in a disordered ear.
Wideband acoustic immittance (WAI)	Evidence is lacking.
Distortion product otoacoustic emissions (DPOAE)	Reduced amplitude or absent at frequencies where there is hearing loss, depending on the degree of hearing
Auditory evoked potentials	N/A
Differential diagnosis	Hemorrhage/aneurysm (due to high vascularization of glomus tumors), otitis media, squamous cell carcinoma, schwannoma, cholesteatoma, otosclerosis, mastoiditis, and osteoma (Pluta & Luliano, 2015)

OSSICULAR FIXATION

Otosclerosis is an alteration of the normal bone remodeling process (Hadjidakis & Androulakis, 2006) that fixes the stapes in place, preventing normal vibration of the ossicular chain, and thus inhibits transfer of energy into the cochlea (NIDCD, 2015). The cause is uncertain and debated, but it appears to have a genetic component. Ossicular fixation is more rarely caused by fibrous adhesions from chronic middle ear infection.

When stimulating an ear with ossicular fixation, expect air-conduction threshold loss up to 60 dB. In contrast, bone conduction thresholds might be normal, resulting in air-bone threshold gaps characteristic of middle ear disorder. However, the air-bone gap caused by ossicular fixation might be minimal or non-existent at 2000 Hz because the fixation alters the normal resonance of the middle ear (Carhart, 1950). This audiometric pattern has been called the Carhart notch.

Fixation surprisingly might have little effect on Y226 Hz tympanograms. Nakajima et al. (2012) reported that ossicular fixation, SSCD, and ossicular discontinuity are the only three disorders that manifest as air-bone gaps on the audiogram in patients with normally aerated middle ears (normal middle ear pressure). However, somewhat similar findings have been reported for patients with large vestibular aqueducts (Attias et al., 2102; Merchant et al., 2007). Narrow widths are possible for Y266, B/G 678 and B/G 1000 Hz tympanograms. The middle ear resonant peak will be higher due to the stiffening effects of the disorder. Acoustic reflex thresholds will be elevated by the amount of the air-bone gap when stimulating a disordered ear and absent when measuring in a disordered ear. Expect OAE to show reduced amplitude or absent depending on the degree of hearing loss and at frequencies where there is hearing loss. For an overview of expectations, see Table 21–4.

TYMPANIC MEMBRANE PERFORATION OR PATENT PRESSURE EQUALIZATION (PE) TUBES

Tympanic membrane (TM) perforations are caused by trauma from foreign object insertion, blows to the head, or barotrauma (Stach, 1998), surgery, or infection. TM perforations due to trauma often heal spontaneously because healthy tissue was present before the injury. However, TM perforations that are caused by infection might not heal naturally if necrosis of the TM had already begun (Martin & Clark, 2015). The location of the TM perforation also has an effect on healing prognosis. TM perforations that involve the outer ring or annulus of the eardrum heal less successfully (Baylor College of Medicine: Otolaryngology-Head and Neck Surgery, n.d). PE tubes are used to treat eustachian tube dysfunction. They function to aerate middle ears, thus taking the place of disordered eustachian tubes in the hope of preventing otitis media.

Table 21–4. Ossicular Fixation

Primary presenting symptom(s)	Gradual hearing loss, family history, paracusis willisii
Otoscopy	Possible Schwartz's sign
Weber tuning fork test	Bone conducted tones might be heard on the affected side in unilateral or asymmetric cases
Pure-tone thresholds	Conductive hearing loss with Carhart notch, but compared to SSCD more hearing loss and larger air-bone gaps from 1000 to 4000 Hz (Nakajima et al., 2012) except at 2000 Hz (see Figure 26–4 in Chapter 26)
WRS	Good to excellent
Y226 Hz tympanometry	Possibly narrow Y226 tympanogram, in only extreme cases lower static admittance
B/G 678 and B/G 1000 Hz tympanometry and middle ear resonance	Narrow 1B1G, B/G 678 and B/G 1000 Hz tympanograms with high resonance frequency
Acoustic reflex thresholds	Acoustic reflex thresholds will be elevated by the amount of the air-bone gap when stimulating a disordered ear and absent when measuring in a disordered ear.
Wideband acoustic immittance (WAI)	Narrow high-frequency reflectance notch at 3000 Hz or above (Feeney, Grant, & Marryott, 2003; Nakajima et al., 2012)
Distortion product otoacoustic emissions (DPOAE)	Reduced amplitude or absent depending on the degree of hearing loss and at frequencies where there is hearing loss

continues

Table 21–4. *continued*

Auditory evoked potentials	N/A
Differential diagnosis	Otitis media, ossicular discontinuity superior semicircular canal dehiscence (SSCD)

Large TM perforations can result in up to a mild conductive hearing loss, while smaller TM perforations might go undetected by the individual (Kramer, 2008). Similarly, patients with PE tubes are unlikely to present with significant hearing loss. If hearing loss does result from TM perforations or patent PE tubes, it will likely manifest as air-bone threshold gaps. Results for Y226 tympanometry will show a large ear canal volume and a flat tracing indicating no changes in admittance during testing. However, tympanometry may not be obtainable due to an inability to maintain a pressure seal; pressure may leak out the Eustachian tube. Acoustic reflex thresholds will be elevated by the amount of the air-bone gap when stimulating a disordered ear and absent when measuring in a disordered ear. Expect OAE amplitude to be reduced or OAE to be absent, depending on the degree of hearing loss and at frequencies where there is hearing loss. For an overview of expectations, see Table 21–5.

Table 21–5. Tympanic Membrane Perforation

Primary presenting symptom(s)	Hollow sensation in the ear, hearing loss, and aural pain or bleeding (Silman & Silverman, 1991)
Otoscopy	Perforation might be visualized, might also see drainage if the perforation is related to infection (Kramer, 2008) or granulation tissue if the perforation is healing (Northern & English, 1991)
Weber tuning fork test	Bone conducted tones likely heard at midline, though they might be heard on the affected side in unilateral or asymmetric cases
Pure-tone thresholds	Ranges from normal hearing to small air-bone gaps (see Figure 26–5 in Chapter 26); total or near total loss of TM can cause greater loss
WRS	Good to excellent
Y226 Hz tympanometry	If a seal can be obtained, expect large ear canal volume and a flat tracing.
B/G678 and 1000 Hz tympanometry	If a seal can be obtained, flat tracing with G greater than B.
Acoustic reflex thresholds	Acoustic reflex thresholds will be elevated by the amount of the air-bone gap when stimulating a disordered ear and absent when measuring in a disordered ear.
Wideband acoustic immittance (WAI)	Decrease in reflectance (trough) in frequencies below 2000 Hz, may be more pronounced as perforation size decreases (Feeney, Grant, & Marryott, 2003; Voss, Merchant, & Horton, 2012)
Distortion product otoacoustic emissions (DPOAE)	Might see reduced amplitude of the lower frequencies when the perforation is small. As perforation size increases, reduced amplitude of the high frequencies will likely be observed (Ueda, Nakata, & Hoshino, 1998).

continues

Table 21–5. *continued*

Auditory evoked potentials	N/A
Vestibular evaluation	When vestibular evaluation is required, proceed with caution; water calorics are contraindicated. Air calorics might yield stronger responses than would be expected if the TM were intact.
Differential diagnosis	Monomer/dimer

MONOMER/DIMER

The tympanic membrane (TM) is comprised of epithelial tissue laterally, fibrous tissue, and mucosal tissue medially. Post trauma or tympanic membrane surgery, all three layers might be restored in the healing process. For some patients, however, the fibrous layer is not restored and the TM is therefore said to be dimeric, consisting only of the epithelial and mucosal layers. If either the epithelial or mucosal layer is also lost, the TM is said to be monomeric (Manolidis, 2003). Otoscopic evaluation is not sufficient to distinguish monomers from dimers, and, therefore, the terms are often used interchangeably (Gopen, 2013).

Monomeric/dimeric TM are unlikely to cause hearing loss unless they are large, then, TM flaccidity might cause a small high frequency conductive loss (Gopen, 2013). Y226 tympanometry might show high admittance, narrow width, and normal ear canal volume (Hunter & Sanford, 2015).Expect B/G 678 and B/G 1000 Hz tympanograms to show multiple peaks (Hunter & Sanford, 2015) with narrow extrema and a low middle ear resonance <75 daPa apart on three-peaked tympanograms and <100 daPa apart on five-peaked tympanograms. Acoustic reflex thresholds should be present at normal levels, unless the hyperflaccidity of the tympanic membrane causes tympanogram tracing fluctuations that obscure measurement. Expect OAE to be normal, although they might be reduced at frequencies where there is an air-bone gap. For an overview of expectations, see Table 21–6.

Table 21–6. Monomer/Dimer

Primary presenting symptom(s)	History of middle ear disease, surgery, or trauma, likely no symptoms associated with the monomer/dimer
Otoscopy	Appearance of a thinning or translucent portion of the TM, may appear to be a perforation (University of Nebraska Medical Center Department of Otolaryngology-Head and Neck Surgery, 2014); often looks dark and can be difficult to differentiate from a perforation; light reflection at center suggests monomer/dimer.
Weber tuning fork test	There will likely be no difference in perception of bone-conducted tones between ears when symmetrical, when there is an asymmetry, the tones will be perceived by the better ear.

continues

Table 21–6. *continued*

Pure-tone thresholds	Monomeric/dimeric TM are unlikely to cause hearing loss, unless they are large, but TM flaccidity might cause a small high frequency conductive loss (Gopen, 2013) (see Figure 26–6 in Chapter 26)
WRS	Good to excellent
Y226 Hz tympanometry	May show high admittance, narrow width, and normal ear canal volume (Hunter & Sanford, 2015).
B/G 678 and B/G 1000 Hz tympanometry and middle ear resonance	Multipeaked B/G 678 and B/G 1000 Hz tympanograms with lateral peaks <75 daPa on the three-peaked tympanogram and <100 daPa on the five-peaked tympanogram. Low resonant frequency (Hunter & Sanford, 2015)
Acoustic reflex thresholds	Likely normal if measureable, the TM flaccidity might manifest as large tracing fluctuations that obscure measurement of acoustic reflexes.
Wideband acoustic immittance (WAI)	Low-frequency trough (Feeney, Grant, & Marryott, 2003)
Distortion product otoacoustic emissions (DPOAE)	OAE are likely to be normal, though they might be reduced at frequencies where there is an air-bone gap.
Auditory evoked potentials	N/A
Differential diagnosis	Perforation, ossicular disarticulation

CHOLESTEATOMA

Cholesteatomas are squamous epithelial cysts composed of keratin debris, which accumulates through desquamation (Dennis & Neely, 1991). Cholesteatomas can be either congenital or acquired, the latter of which can be further divided into primary and secondary cases. Primary acquired is the most commonly occurring form of cholesteatoma (Barátha, Huberb, Stämpflid, Vargac, & Kollias, 2011). They arise when the TM is retracted due to middle ear disorder (Olszewska et al., 2004), and epithelial cells become trapped in the retraction pocket (Gopen, 2013). Secondary acquired cholesteatoma is often associated with middle ear disorder (Olszewska et al., 2004) and is the product of epithelial cells that have been introduced into the middle ear space via either a perforation or as a remnant of otologic surgery (e.g. the placement of PE tubes; Gopen, 2013). Perforation of the pars flaccida or posterior superior quadrant of the TM opens the possibility of acquired cholesteatoma in that region of the middle ear space (Gopen, 2013; Silman & Silverman, 1991; Weber, 2007). Acquired middle ear cholesteatomas have a slightly higher prevalence in males than females and are more likely to be diagnosed in individuals under the age of 50 (Barátha et al., 2011).

Congenital cholesteatomas are rare, accounting for approximately 5% of all cases (Paparella & Rybak, 1978). Approximately 75% of congenital cholesteatomas occur in the anterosuperior quadrant of the middle ear space (Potsic, Samadi, Marsh, & Wetmore, 2002), and are characterized by a normal tympanic membrane with no previous history of middle ear pathology. They are diagnosed almost exclusively in children (Weber, 2007).

When stimulating an ear with cholesteatoma, expect air conduction threshold loss up to 60 dB. Bone conduction thresholds will be normal, yielding an air-bone threshold gap. If the cholesteatoma invades the cochlea, a mixed hearing loss will result. Cholesteatoma might manifest as lower Y226 Hz static admittance with wide or even flat widths. Acoustic reflex thresholds will likely be elevated when stimulating an ear with a cholesteatoma and absent when measuring reflexes in that same ear. Expect OAE to be reduced amplitude or absent, depending on the degree of hearing loss and at frequencies where there is hearing loss. For an overview of expectations, see Table 21–7.

Table 21–7. Cholesteatoma

Primary presenting symptom(s)	Aural pain, tinnitus, foul smelling discharge, hearing loss (Silman & Silverman, 1991), and history of middle ear infection (Olszewska et al., 2004)
Otoscopy	White or pearly mass and/or granulation tissue behind the TM or within a retraction pocket and perforation of the pars flaccida or posterior superior quadrant of the TM where acquired cholesteatoma are often seen (Gopen, 2013; Silman & Silverman, 1991; Weber, 2007). Approximately 75% of congenital cholesteatomas occur in the anterosuperior quadrant of the middle ear space (Potsic, Samadi, Marsh, & Wetmore, 2002).
Weber tuning fork test	Bone conducted tones might be heard on the affected side in unilateral or asymmetric cases

Table 21–7. *continued*

Pure-tone thresholds	Conductive hearing loss, a sensorineural component may be present if cholesteatoma has invaded the inner ear (see Figure 26–7 in Chapter 26)
WRS	Good to excellent if solely a conductive impairment, can be poorer if a mixed hearing loss is present
Y226 Hz tympanometry	Low- to no-admittance, wide width, and normal ear canal volume (Hunter & Sanford, 2015)
B/G 678 and B/G 1000 Hz tympanometry and resonant peak	B/G 678 and B/G 1000 Hz tympanometry may be wide or flat with B higher than G (Fowler, 2002). Resonant peak will likely be low (Hunter & Sanford, 2015).
Acoustic reflex thresholds	Acoustic reflex thresholds will be elevated by the amount of the air-bone gap when stimulating a disordered ear and absent when measuring in a disordered ear.
Wideband acoustic immittance (WAI)	Data are unavailable, although generally higher reflectance (lower absorbance) is expected. Stiffening of middle ear could shift trough to higher frequencies, added mass or TM perforation could shift trough to lower frequencies.
Distortion product otoacoustic emissions (DPOAE)	Reduced amplitude or absent depending on the degree of hearing loss and at frequencies where there is hearing loss
Auditory evoked potentials	N/A
Differential diagnosis	Cholesterol granulomas, glomus tumors, facial nerve hemangiomas (Barátha, Huberb, Stämpflid, Vargac, & Kollias, 2011)

CERUMEN

Cerumen and oil are secreted from glands in the outer one-third of the ear canal. Cerumen serves to protect the ear by trapping dirt, debris, and insects, and it has minor antibacterial properties. Oil lubricates the skin. Ear "wax" is a combination of cerumen, oil, dirt, hair, debris, and microorganisms. Symptoms might include hearing loss, fullness or plugged feeling, otalgia, itchiness, odor or other discharge, tinnitus, and even dizziness. In most cases, ear canals are self-cleaning by a slow outward migration of skin cells that moves earwax laterally, as on a conveyor belt. That migration can be reversed by use of cotton-tipped ear cleaners or even hearing aids. Cerumen occlusions of as little as 40% of the ear canal diameter can cause minimal hearing loss of 5 to 15 dB, whereas 100% occlusions can cause hearing loss of 40 dB or more (Roeser, Lai, & Clark, 2005). The audiogram will show abnormal air conduction thresholds but normal bone conduction thresholds, though small bone-conduction shifts are possible when cerumen has "loaded" the tympanic membrane (Tonndorf, 1968). Acoustic reflex thresholds will be elevated by the amount of the air-bone gap when stimulating a disordered ear and absent when measuring in a disordered ear. Expect OAE amplitude to be reduced or absent depending on the degree of hearing loss and at frequencies where there is hearing loss. For an overview of expectations, see Table 21–8.

Table 21–8. Cerumen

Primary presenting symptom(s)	Hearing loss, fullness or plugged feeling, otalgia, itchiness, odor or other discharge, tinnitus, and even dizziness
Otoscopy	Cerumen impaction or occlusion
Weber tuning fork test	Bone conducted tones might be heard on the affected side in unilateral or asymmetric cases
Pure-tone thresholds	Conductive hearing loss, possible bone conduction notch at 1000 Hz or more rarely at 2000 (see Figure 26–8 in Chapter 26)
WRS	Good to excellent
Y226 Hz tympanometry	Flat with low physical (ear canal) volume
B/G 678 and B/G 1000 Hz tympanometry	Flat with B greater than G
Acoustic reflex thresholds	Acoustic reflex thresholds will be elevated by the amount of the air-bone gap when stimulating a disordered ear and absent when measuring in a disordered ear.
Wideband acoustic immittance (WAI)	N/A
Distortion product otoacoustic emissions (DPOAE)	Reduced amplitude or absent depending on the degree of hearing loss and at frequencies where there is hearing loss
Auditory evoked potentials	N/A
Differential diagnosis	Perforation or PE tube, otitis media

REFERENCES

Attias J, Ulanovski D. Shemesh, R., Kornreich, L., Nageris, B., Preis, M., . . . Raveh, E. (2012). Air-bone gap component of inner-ear origin in audiograms of cochlear implant candidates. *Otology & Neurotology*, *33*, 512–L517.

Barátha, K., Huberb, A., Stämpflid, P., Vargac, Z, & Kollias, S. (2011). Neuroradiology of cholesteatomas. *American Journal of Neuroradiology*, *32*, 221–229.

Baylor College of Medicine Otolaryngology-Head and Neck Surgery. (n.d). *Tympanic membrane perforation*. Retrieved from https://www.bcm.edu/healthcare/care-centers/otolaryngology/conditions/tympanic-membrane-perforation

Carhart, R. (1950). Clinical application of bone conduction audiometry. *Archives of Otolaryngology*, *51*, 798–808.

Dennis, J. M., & Neely, J.G. (1991). Otoneurologic diseases and associated audiologic profiles. In J. T. Jacobson & J. L. Northern (Eds.), *Diagnostic audiology* (pp. 83–109). Austin, TX: Pro-Ed.

Feeney, M. P., Grant, I. L., & Marryott, L. P. (2003). Wideband energy reflectance measurements in adults with middle-ear disorders. *Journal of Speech Language and Hearing Research*, *46*, 901–911.

Gopen, Q. (2013). *Fundamental otology: Pediatric and adult practice*. New Delhi, India: Jaypee Brothers Medical.

Hadjidakis, D. J., & Androulakis, I. I. (2006). Bone remodeling. *Annals of the New York Academy of Science*, *1092*, 385–396. Retrieved from http://www.ncbi.nlm.nih.gov/pubmed/17308163

Hall, J. W., III, & Ghorayeb, B. Y. (1991). Diagnosis of middle ear pathology and evaluation of conductive hearing loss. In J. T. Jacobson & J. L. Northern (Eds.), *Diagnostic audiology* (p. 161–198). Austin, TX: Pro-Ed.

Harris, P.K., Hutchinson, K. M., & Moravec, J. (2005). The use of tympanometry and pneumatic otoscopy for predicting middle ear disease. *American Journal of Audiology, 14*, 3–13.

Hunter, L. L., & Sanford, C. A. (2015). Tympanometry and wideband acoustic immitance. In J. Katz, M. Chasin, K. English, L. Hood, & K. Tillery (Eds.), *Handbook of clinical audiology* (7th ed., pp. 137–161). Philadelphia, PA: Wolters Kluwer.

Jerger, S., & Jerger, J. (1981). *Auditory disorders: A manual for clinical evaluation*. Boston, MA: Little, Brown.

Kramer, S. (2008). *Audiology: Science to practice*. San Diego, CA: Plural.

Kumar, M., Maheshwar, A., Mahendran, S., Oluwasamni, A., & Clayton, M. I. (2003). Could the presence of a Carhart notch predict the presence of glue at myringotomy? *Clinical Otolaryngology, 28*(3), 183–186.

Manolidis, S. (2003). Closure of tympanic membrane perforations. In M. Glasscock III & A. Gulya (Eds.), *Glasscock-Shambaugh: Surgery of the ear* (5th ed., pp. 400–419). Hamilton, Ontario: B.C. Decker.

Martin, F. & Clark, J. G. (2015). *Introduction to audiology*. Boston, MA: Pearson.

Merchant S. N., Rosowski J. J., & McKenna M. J. (2007). Superior semicircular canal dehiscence mimicking otosclerotic hearing loss. *Advances in Oto-Rhino-Laryngology, 65*, 137–145.

Nakajima, H. H., Pisano, D. V., Roosli, C., Hamade, M. A., Merchant, G. R., Mahfood, L., . . . Merchant, S. N. (2012). Comparison of ear-canal reflectance and umbo velocity in patients with conductive hearing loss: A preliminary study. *Ear and Hearing, 33*(1), 35–43.

National Institute on Deafness and Other Communication Disorders. (2015). *Otosclerosis*. Retrieved from http://www.nidcd.nih.gov/health/hearing/Pages/otosclerosis.aspx

Olszewska, E., Wagner, M., Bernal-Sprekelsen, M., Ebmeyer, J., Dazert, S., Hildmann, H., & Sudhoff, H. (2004). Etiopathogenesis of cholesteatoma. *European Archives of Oto-Rhino-Laryngology, 261*, 6–24.

Paparella, M. M., Morizono, T., Le, C. T., Mancini, F., Sipilä, P., Choo, . . . Ki, C. S. (1984). Sensory-neural hearing loss in otitis media. *Annals of Otology, Rhinology, and Laryngology, 93*, 623–629.

Paparella, M. M., & Rybak, L. (1978). Congenital cholesteatoma, *Otolaryngolic Clinics of North America, 11*(1), 113–120.

Pluta, R., & Iuliano, B. (2015). *Glomus tumors*. Retrieved from http://emedicine.medscape.com/ article/ 251009 –overview

Potsic, W. P., Samadi, D. S., Marsh, R. R., & Wetmore, R. F. (2002). A staging system for congenital cholesteatoma. *Archives of Otolaryngology-Head and Neck Surgery, 128*(9), 1009–1012.

Roeser, R.J., Lai, L., & Clark, J.L. (2005). Effect of ear canal occlusion on pure-tone threshold sensitivity. *Journal of the American Academy of Audiology, 16*(9), 740–746.

Sautter, N., & Hirose, K., (2007). Otitis media. In G. B. Hughes & M. L. Pensak (Eds.), *Clinical otology* (pp. 223–233). New York, NY: Thieme Medical.

Silman, S., & Silverman, C. (1991). *Auditory diagnosis: Principles and applications.* San Diego, CA: Academic Press.

Stach, B. A. (1998). *Clinical audiology.* San Diego, CA: Singular.

Tonndorf, J., (1968). A new concept of bone conduction. *Archives of Otolaryngology, 87*, 49–54.

Ueda, H., Nakata, S., & Hoshino, M. (1998). Effects of effusion in the middle ear and perforation of the tympanic membrane on optoacoustic emissions in guinea pigs. *Hearing Research, 122*(1–2), 41–46.

University of Nebraska Medical Center Department of Otolaryngology-Head and Neck Surgery. (2014). *Unit five: Tympanic membrane perforations.* Retrieved from http://app1.unmc.edu/ medicine/heywood/otology/unit5-tympanic-membrane-perforations.cfm

Weber, P. (2007). Chronic otitis media. In G. B. Hughes & M. L. Pensak (Eds.), *Clinical otology* (pp. 236–249). New York, NY: Thieme.

Wiley, T. L., Oviatt, D. L., & Block, M. G. J. (1987). Acoustic-immittance measures in normal ears. *Journal of Speech and Hearing Research*, *38*, 490–502.

Yasan, H. (2007). Predictive role of Carhart's notch in pre-operative assessment for middle-ear surgery. *Journal of Laryngology and Otology*, *121*, 219–221.

22

Inner Ear Disorders

NOISE-INDUCED HEARING LOSS

Noise-induced hearing loss (NIHL) occurs as a result of occupational, recreational, or accidental noise exposures. Intense sound can damage cochlear hair cells, including cell membranes or stereocillia, hair cell metabolic exhaustion, and neural excitotoxicity (Kujawa & Liberman, 2009; Schlauch & Nelson, 2015), and even damage to supporting cells and membranes. Tinnitus and hyperacusis can also be reported (Fligor, Chasin, & Neitzel, 2015). A NIHL can occur in individuals of any age and, according to the National Institute on Deafness and Other Communication Disorders (NIDCD), (2014), 15 to 20% of individuals aged 12 to 69 years have reported experiencing hearing loss that may have been due to noise exposure. Generally, the greater the sound intensity, the shorter the duration that intense noise can be tolerated without risk of hearing loss (NIDCD, 2014). However, NIHL is influenced by individual variability, including genetics.

Noise exposure can cause permanent hearing loss (permanent threshold shift, or PTS) or temporary hearing loss (temporary threshold shift, or TTS). TTS manifests as a worsening of hearing thresholds that recover, often within 48 hours of the noise exposure. However, TTS does not preclude insidious permanent neural damage (Kujawa & Liberman, 2009).

For patients with NIHL, air conduction and bone conduction thresholds will be similar and often show a notch defined as greater hearing loss at 3000 Hz, 4000 Hz, or 6000 Hz, compared to thresholds at surrounding test frequencies (Lundborg, 1980; Schlauch & Nelson, 2015). Initially, hearing loss will likely be symmetric between ears, however, asymmetric NIHL can occur in instances when the individual has been exposed to greater amounts of noise on one side of the body (Rabinowitz, 2000). Common examples include right-handed rifle fire, exposing the left ear to noise from the barrel, or a factory worker standing to the right of a noisy machine. In these two examples, the left ear might show greater hearing loss.

A NIHL will manifest as a sensorineural hearing loss; air and bone conduction thresholds should be in agreement. In cases where NIHL affects primarily outer hair cells, a maximum of approximately 60 dB hearing loss will be measured at any given pure-tone test frequency. Hearing loss greater than 60 dB suggests concomitant inner hair cell damage. Neural damage can occur regardless of hair cell involvement.

Admittance tympanometry with a 226 Hz probe tone (Y226) will yield results within normal limits. At disordered frequencies acoustic reflex thresholds will be present at low sensation levels (≤60 dBSL) when inner hair cells are intact and elevated or absent when inner hair cells are damaged. Otoacoustic emissions (OAE) will be at reduced amplitude or absent when testing affected frequencies. Auditory brainstem response (ABR) evaluation will be variable depending on degree of loss and extent of concomitant neural disorder. For an overview of expectations, see Table 22–1.

Table 22–1. Noise-Induced Hearing Loss

Primary presenting symptom(s)	Hearing loss, tinnitus, hyperacusis (Fligor, Chasin, & Neitzel, 2015)
Otoscopy	Normal
Weber tuning fork test	Tone would be heard at midline for symmetric hearing loss. For asymmetrical hearing losses, if testing at a disordered frequency, tones will be heard in the better ear.
Pure-tone thresholds	Expect high frequency sensorineural hearing loss, often initially notched in the 3000 to 6000 Hz range; degree of loss is dependent on intensity and duration of noise exposure. (Figure 26–9, Chapter 26)
WRS	Good unless inner hair cells and neurons are significantly damaged (McArdle & Hnath-Chisolm, 2015)
Y226 Hz tympanometry	Within normal limits
B/G 678 and B/G 1000 Hz tympanometry and middle ear resonance	Within normal limits
Acoustic reflex thresholds	Low sensation with outer hair cell damage only, elevated or absent when inner hair cells are damaged
Wideband acoustic immittance (WAI)	Within normal limits
Distortion product otoacoustic emissions (DPOAE)	Reduced amplitude or absent at affected frequencies

continues

Table 22–1. *continued*

Auditory evoked potentials	Consistent with audiometric thresholds
Differential diagnosis	Presbycusis, autoimmune disease of the inner ear, genetic sensorineural hearing loss, ototoxicity (Mathur & Roland, 2014)

PRESBYCUSIS

Presbycusis is gradually progressive hearing loss, typically bilaterally, related to the process of aging (NIDCD, 2013). Presbycusis sites of lesion can be sensory, neural, strial, and cochlear conductive (Schuknecht & Gacek, 1993). Each type has characteristic signs and symptoms that will be reviewed separately below. However, it is important for the audiologist to remember that the different presbycusis types can occur in combination.

Sensory presbycusis results from atrophy of the organ of Corti, including degeneration of supporting cells and hair cells (primarily outer hair cells). Damage is typically worse in the basal portion of the cochlea (Weinstein, 2015). Damage to these structures begins near the end of middle- age and progresses slowly over time (Roland, 2015). Sensory presbycusis is characterized by a precipitously sloping high-frequency sensorineural hearing loss;

speech understanding therefore, is relatively preserved (Roland, 2015).

Neural presbycusis involves degradation of auditory neurons. We lose approximately 2,000 or more neurons every decade of life, but symptoms manifest only later in life when the neuron population has dropped below a minimum level (Suzuka & Schuknecht, 1988). Speech understanding can be affected (Gaeth, 1948), but approximately 90% of neurons must be lost before audiometric thresholds are affected (Roland, 2015). Neuron loss is typically greatest among the neurons innervating the basal end of the cochlea.

Strial presbycusis is caused by atrophy of the stria vascularis, which can begin as early as the third decade of life (Roland, 2015). Damage to the stria vascularis can affect endolymph production and regulation, which can impact hair cell function from base to apex (Roland, 2015; Schuknecht, 1964). Accordingly, strial presbycusis manifests as a slowly progressing sensorineural hearing loss with a relatively flat audiometric pattern with speech understanding largely preserved.

Cochlear conductive presbycusis, also known as mechanical presbycusis, results from the widening and stiffening of the base of the basilar membrane by calcification (Schuknecht, 1964). This affects traveling wave motion and causes a gradually sloping high frequency sensorineural hearing loss, with speech understanding largely preserved (Roland, 2015).

All types of presbycusis manifest as a sensorineural hearing loss; air and bone condution thresholds should be in agreement. The degree and slope of the loss will be dependent on site of lesion and the degree of damage. Damage to outer hair cells can result in a maximum of approximately 60-dB hearing loss at any given pure-tone test frequency. Hearing loss greater than 60 dB suggests concomitant inner hair cell damage.

Y226 tympanometry results will be within normal limits. At disordered frequencies, acoustic reflex thresholds will be present at low sensation levels (≤60 dBSL) when inner hair cells are intact, and elevated or absent when inner hair cells are damaged. OAE's will be at reduced amplitude or absent when testing affected frequencies. ABR evaluation will be variable depending on degree of loss and extent of concomitant neural disorder. For an overview of expectations see Table 22–2.

Table 22–2. Presbycusis

Primary presenting symptom(s)	Hearing loss, difficulty differentiating between high frequency speech sounds (e.g., consonants), speech may sound mumbled or slurred, difficulty understanding speech in noise (NIDCD, 2013)
Otoscopy	Within normal limits
Weber tuning fork test	Tone is heard at midline for symmetric hearing loss. For asymmetrical hearing losses, if testing at a disordered frequency, tones will be heard in the better ear.

Table 22–2. *continued*

Pure-tone thresholds	Sensorineural hearing loss with configuration dependent upon the type(s) of presbycusis involved. The configuration could be sloping, flat-to-sloping, or with a precipitous high-frequency drop. (Figure 26–10, Chapter 26)
WRS	Good with outer hair cell disorder, poorer with involvement of inner hair cells and neurons.
Y226 Hz tympanometry	Within normal limits
B/G 678 and B/G 1000 Hz tympanometry and middle ear resonance	Within normal limits
Acoustic reflex thresholds	Low sensation level with outer hair cell damage only, elevated or absent when inner hair cells are damaged.
Wideband acoustic immittance (WAI)	Within normal limits
Distortion product otoacoustic emissions (DPOAE)	Reduced amplitude or absent at affected frequencies
Auditory evoked potentials	Consistent with audiometric thresholds
Differential diagnosis	Noise-induced hearing loss

SUPERIOR SEMICIRCULAR CANAL DEHISCENCE (SSCD)

Superior semicircular canal dehiscence (SSCD) is a thinning or absence of the temporal bone at the semicircular canal superiorly, which uncovers the membranous inner-ear labyrinth within. This creates a third membranous window, the first two being the oval and round windows.

When stimulating an ear with SSCD, air conduction thresholds might show hearing loss; air-conducted energy might be shunted out of the dehiscence. In contrast, bone conduction thresholds might be normal or even better than expected; bone-conducted energy might enter the cochlea through the dehiscence. The resulting air-bone gap in these patients has been called a conductive or mixed hearing loss (Chien, Janky, Minor, & Carey, 2012), but these terms might best be reserved for patients with hearing loss from outer or middle ear disorder. An SSCD is an inner ear disorder, and therefore the term "air-bone gaps of inner ear origin" might be more precise (Attias et al., 2012). The air-bone gaps are typically seen in the lower test frequencies (Nakajima, et al, 2012). Symptoms of SSCD include: low frequency hearing loss (Minor, 2005), pulsatile tinnitus, autophony and audition of other body noises, dizziness, oscillopsia, pressure-induced (coughing, sneezing, straining) symptoms, Tullio phenomenon, and Hennebert sign (Minor, 2005).

Nakajima et al. (2012) reported that SSCD, ossicular fixation, and ossicular discontinuity are the only three disorders that manifest as air-bone gaps on the audiogram in patients with normally aerated middle ears, though somewhat similar findings have been reported for patients with large vestibular aqueducts (Attias et al., 2102; Merchant, Rosowski & McKenna, 2007). With SSCD, normally aerated middle ears can be confirmed with Y226 Hz tympanometry, though larger static admittance might be seen on the affected side (Castellucci, Brandolini, Piras, & Modugno, 2013). The reason for this might be due to the opening of a third cochlear window, which could lower inner ear pressure. Lower middle ear resonance can be measured because the middle ear interfaces with the inner ear (Bilgen, Kirkim & Kirazli,2009; Rosowski et al., 2004; Sato et al., 2002). Both B/G 678 Hz and B/G 1000 tympanograms should show <5B peaks and/or <3G. Acoustic reflexes will be present, unlike cases of ossicular fixation and ossicular discontinuity. OAE might be largely present as well, assuming no hair cell damage. For an overview of expectations, see Table 22–3.

Table 22–3. Superior Semicircular Canal Dehiscence (SSCD)

Primary presenting symptom(s)	Low frequency hearing loss (Minor, 2005), pulsatile tinnitus, autophony and audition of other body noises, dizziness, oscillopsia, pressure-induced (coughing, sneezing, straining) symptoms, Tullio phenomenon, Hennebert sign (Minor, 2005)
Otoscopy	Normal
Weber tuning fork test	Bone conducted tones might be heard on the affected side (Minor, 2005).
Pure-tone thresholds	Low-frequency hearing loss with air-bone threshold gaps of inner-ear origin, mimicking conductive or mixed hearing loss (Figure 26–11, Chapter 26)

continues

Table 22–3. *continued*

WRS	Good to excellent
Y226 Hz tympanometry	Within normal limits, possibly with greater static compliance on the affected ear
B/G 678 Hz and B/G 1000 Hz tympanometry and middle ear resonance	Expect results to be generally within normal limits. However, a lower resonant frequency appears possible based on reports of lower resonant frequencies associated with another third window pathology, large vestibular aqueducts (Bilgen et al., 2009; Rosowski, et al., 2004; Sato et al., 2002).
Acoustic reflex thresholds	Present
Wideband acoustic immittance (WAI)	WAI can appear somewhat normal but with less reflectance at 1000 Hz (Nakajima et al., 2012), or it can show a multipeaked WAI pattern with a primary low-frequency trough similar to tympanic membrane pathology, tympanic membrane perforations, and ossicular disarticulations.
Distortion product otoacoustic emissions (DPOAE)	Largely present
Auditory evoked potentials	Consistent with audiometric thresholds
Vestibular evaluation	Low VEMP thresholds on the affected side (Minor, 2005)
Differential diagnosis	Otitis media, ossicular fixation, ossicular discontinuity

LARGE VESTIBULAR AQUEDUCT

Large vestibular aqueduct (LVA) might manifest as hearing loss early in life and have insidious onset, or it might be associated with barotrauma or other traumas. A LVA causes sensory/neural hearing loss (Attias et al., 2012; Jackler & De La Cruz, 1989; Mimura et al., 2005). The cause of the sensory/neural hearing loss component is unclear. It may result from increased endolymph pressure from the endolymphatic duct and sac that damages hair cells, or by endolymph electrolyte changes that are harmful to the hair cells or stria vascularis (Campbell, Adunka, Zhou, Qaqish, & Buchman, 2011; Jackler & De La Cruz, 1989; Levinson, Parisier, Jacobs, & Edelstein, 1989). In addition, LVA also opens a third window, the first two being the oval and round windows. Air-bone gaps are therefore possible as air-conduction thresholds might be lowered (made poorer) because air-conducted energy is shunted away from the cochlea through the LVA, whereas bone-conduction thresholds might be improved by sound pressure transmissions through the skull contents, and in turn through the LVA. The air-bone gap in these patients has been called a conductive or mixed hearing loss (Chien, Janky, Minor, & Carey, 2012); terms perhaps best reserved for patients with middle ear disorder. The term air-bone gaps of inner ear origin might be more appropriate (Attias et al., 2012).

When stimulating an ear with an LVA, expect air-conduction and bone-conduction thresholds to be reduced compared to normal due to sensory/neural disorder, but with air-bone gaps as described above. Expect normal Y226 Hz tympanometry; LVA might be one of a few disorders that manifest as air-bone gaps on the audiogram in patients with normally aerated middle ears (Attias et al., 2102; Merchant et al., 2007). Other disorders that might manifest as similar patterns include SSCD, ossicular fixation and ossicular discontinuity (Nakajima et al., 2012). Both B/G 678 Hz and B/G 1000 tympano-grams should show ≤5B peaks and/or ≤3G. However, the third window could lower cochlear pressure. Lower middle ear resonance can be measured because the middle ear interfaces with the inner ear (Bilgen et al., 2009; Rosowski et al., 2004; Sato et al., 2002). At disordered frequencies, acoustic reflex thresholds will be present at low sensation levels (≤60 dB SL) when inner hair cells are intact, and elevated or absent when inner hair cells are damaged. OAE's will be at reduc-ed amplitude or absent when testing affected frequencies. ABR evaluation will be variable, depending on degree of loss and extent of concomitant neural disorder. For an overview of expectations see Table 22–4.

Table 22–4. Large Vestibular Aqueduct

Primary presenting symptom(s)	Symptoms include hearing loss that might manifest early in life and have insidious onset; or it might be associated with barotrauma or other traumas.
Otoscopy	Normal
Weber tuning fork test	Tone is heard at midline for symmetric hearing loss. For asymmetrical hearing losses, if testing at a disordered frequency, tones will be heard in the better ear.

Table 22–4. *continued*

Pure-tone thresholds	Sensory/neural hearing loss with air-bone gaps of inner ear origin mimicking conductive or mixed hearing loss (Figure 26–12, Chapter 26)
WRS	Variable depending on the degree of sensory/neural hearing loss
Y226 Hz tympanometry	Within normal limits
B/G 678 and B/G 1000 Hz tympanometry and middle ear resonance	B/G 678 Hz and B/G 1000 tympanograms should show <5B peaks and/or <3G, but resonant frequency might be low (Sato et al., 2002)
Acoustic reflex thresholds	Low sensation level with outer hair cell damage only, elevated or absent when inner hair cells are damaged
Wideband acoustic immittance (WAI)	No data available
Distortion product otoacoustic emissions (DPOAE)	Reduced amplitude or absent at affected frequencies
Auditory evoked potentials	Consistent with audiometric thresholds
Vestibular evaluation	Low VEMP thresholds on the affected side (Minor, 2005)
Differential diagnosis	Superior semicircular canal dehiscence

OTOTOXICITY

Some prescription drugs are ototoxic, most commonly cochleotoxic, but sometimes vestibulotoxic (American Academy of Audiology (AAA, 2009). The most common ototoxic drugs encountered in audiology practice and elsewhere are aminoglycosides, platinum coordination complexes, loop diuretics, and nonsteroidal anti-inflammatory drugs (Humes, 1999; Garcia et al., 2001). The risk of otoxicity and severity of outcomes depend on several factors including, the drug administered, the dose, liver and kidney disorder affecting drug excretion, patient age, and cardiac health.

Ototoxicity will manifest as a sensorineural hearing loss; air and bone conduction thresholds should be in agreement. Hearing loss will typically manifest first at higher test frequencies above 8000 Hz (Schlauch & Nelson, 2015; Fausti et al., 1992). However, audiologists should be vigilant because mid-frequency ototoxic hearing loss is possible (AAA, 2009).

Y226 tympanometry results will be within normal limits. Acoustic reflex thresholds will be measured at low sensation levels (<60 dB SL) at frequencies where hearing loss is present, and is due to outer hair cell disorder. At frequencies where inner hair cell disorder has occurred, the hearing loss will be worse and the acoustic reflex thresholds will be elevated or absent. OAEs will be reduced in amplitude or absent at frequencies where outer hair cell damage has occurred. As a caveat, audiologists should recall that at least one ototoxic drug, Carboplatin, might primarily damage inner hair cells (Lobarinas, Salvi, & Ding, 2013). This could manifest as normal OAE, hearing loss, and elevated or absent acoustic reflexes.

The American Academy of Audiology published a position statement on ototoxicity monitoring (2009). The details of that position statement are beyond the scope of this text, but salient aspects are offered here. When practical, a baseline audiologic evaluation should be performed before any ototoxic drugs have been administered so that ototoxicity can be differentiated from pre-existing hearing loss. However, aminoglycoside ototoxicity typically begins up to 72 hours post administration, so a baseline evaluation can be considered valid within approximately 48 hours of first drug administration. The baseline should be comprehensive so that the audiologist can differentiate sensorineural hearing loss from unrelated conductive hearing loss, and allow for treatment for hearing loss affecting communication. To those ends, a baseline evaluation should include air and bone conduction thresholds, high-frequency air conduction thresholds (some audiometers can generate frequencies as high as 22,000 Hz), word recognition scores, immittance, and otoacoustic emissions.

Often, the most important test for ototoxic monitoring is high-frequency air conduction audiometry; standard frequency audiometry is sufficient for patients who cannot hear higher frequencies due to pre-existing hearing loss. The AAA ototoxicity guideline authors recommended a shortened serial monitoring protocol; identify at baseline the highest frequency above 8000 Hz at which a 100 dB SPL threshold was measured, and monitor that frequency plus the next six lower frequencies in 1/6th octave steps (or the next six lower frequencies available on the audiometer). If there is no hearing above 8000 Hz, identify the highest frequency at which a 100-dB HL threshold was measured and monitor that frequency plus the next six lower frequencies in

1/6th octave steps (or the next six lower frequencies available on the audiometer). The American Speech-Language Hearing Association's (1994) significant change criteria can be used to compare a monitoring audiogram to the baseline audiogram:

- >20 dB decrease at any one test frequency (relative to baseline)
- >10 dB decrease at any two or more adjacent frequencies (relative to baseline)
- Loss of response at three consecutive frequencies where responses were previously obtained (relative to baseline)

Change should be confirmed by retest within 24 hours. Some patients being treated with ototoxic drugs have significant illness precluding participation in standard audiometrics, either at baseline or monitoring. In such cases, distortion product otoacoustic emissions (DPOAE) should be considered. If DPOAE are present at baseline, they can be used for monitoring. We recommend change criteria of >6 dB DPOAE amplitude change, or loss of response at two consecutive frequencies (Dille et al., 2010).

Monitoring for aminoglycoside ototoxicity should be conducted at least bi-weekly, and continue a few months after cessation of the drug to allow for drug clearance by excretion. Monitoring for platinum-based chemotherapy should occur prior to each treatment, and continue a few months after cessation of the drug, or up to 2 years after cessation of the drug if treatment included head and neck radiation. Noise exposure should be avoided for some time post treatment, as these patients might be more susceptible to NIHL (American Academy of Audiology, 2009). For an overview of expectations see Table 22–5.

Table 22–5. Ototoxicity

Primary presenting symptom(s)	Hearing loss, vertigo, nausea, gait instability, and tinnitus preceding loss of hearing sensitivity (American Academy of Audiology, 2009)
Otoscopy	Within normal limits
Weber tuning fork test	Tone is heard at midline for symmetric hearing loss. For asymmetrical hearing losses, if testing at a disordered frequency, tones will be heard in the better ear.
Pure-tone thresholds	High frequency sensorineural hearing loss, including above 8000 Hz if testable; degree of loss is variable (Figure 26–13, Chapter 26)
WRS	If damage is confined to the outer hair cells, WRS can be relatively good, however, with inner hair cell involvement WRS is normally very poor (McArdle & Hnath-Chisolm, 2015).
Y226 Hz tympanometry	Within normal limits
B/G 678 and B/G 1000 Hz tympanometry and middle ear resonance	Within normal limits
Acoustic reflex thresholds	Low sensation level with outer hair cell damage only, elevated or absent when inner hair cells are damaged
Wideband acoustic immittance (WAI)	Within normal limits
Distortion product otoacoustic emissions (DPOAE)	Expect reduced amplitude or absent at affected frequencies when damage occurs to the outer hair cells. In rarer cases in which damage is primarily localized to the inner hair cells, results will likely be normal.

continues

Table 22–5. *continued*

Auditory evoked potentials	Consistent with audiometric thresholds
Vestibular evaluation	Peripheral abnormality
Differential diagnosis	Ménière's disease, noise-induced hearing loss, presbycusis, sudden sensorineural hearing loss, acoustic neuroma/vestibular schwannoma, labyrinthitis

INNER EAR INFECTION

Both viral and bacterial types of infections have been associated with sensorineural hearing loss of both insidious and sudden onset, often with vestibular symptoms. Viral infections implicated in sensorineural hearing loss include cytomegalovirus (CMV), rubeola (measles), mumps, rubella, herpes simplex, varicella zoster, Epstein-Barr, hepatitis, variola, adenovirus, influenza, parainfluenza, polio, encephalitis, infectious mononucleosis, and human immunodeficiency virus (Gates, 2000; Monsell et al., 2007). Bacterial infections implicated in sensorineural hearing loss include bacterial meningitis, syphilis, and Lyme disease (Berlow, Caldarelli, Matz, Meyer, & Harsch, 1980; Dobbin & Perkins, 1983; Peltomaa, Pyykko, Seppälä, Viitanen, & Viljanen, 2000). Middle ear infections such as otitis media might also have the potential to spread to the inner ear and cause sensorineural hearing loss if left untreated (Paparella et al., 1984).

Pure-tone air and bone conduction thresholds should be in agreement and reveal a sensorineural hearing loss that is often unilateral (Gates, 2000). Y226 tympanometry results will likely be within normal limits unless a conductive disorder is also present. Acoustic reflexes thresholds will be at low sensation levels (<60 dBSL) if only outer hair cells are affected, but elevated or absent if inner hair cells are affected. Similarly, DPOAE's will be reduced or absent at frequencies in which there is outer hair cell damage. For an overview of expectations see Table 22–6.

Table 22–6. Inner Ear Infection

Primary presenting symptom(s)	Sudden onset hearing loss, severe loss of hearing and/or vestibular function, and lack of spontaneous recovery would occur in most cases (Gates, 2000). Exceptions include syphilis and Lyme disease, in which recovery from sudden SNHL is possible with proper treatment (Balkany & Dans, 1978; Hanner, Rosenhall, Edstrom, & Kaijser, 1989).
Otoscopy	Within normal limits
Weber tuning fork test	Tone is heard at midline for symmetric hearing loss. For asymmetrical hearing losses, if testing at a disordered frequency, tones will be heard in the better ear.
Pure-tone thresholds	Often unilateral sudden sensorineural hearing loss (Figure 26–14, Chapter 26)
WRS	If damage is confined to the outer hair cells, WRS can be good, however, with inner hair cell involvement, WRS is poorer (McArdle & Hnath-Chisolm, 2015).

continues

Table 22–6. *continued*

Y226 Hz tympanometry	Within normal limits
B/G 678 and B/G 1000 Hz tympanometry and middle ear resonance	Within normal limits
Acoustic reflexes	Expect low sensation level, (<60 dB SL), with outer hair cell damage only, elevated or absent when inner hair cells are damaged.
Wideband acoustic immittance (WAI)	Within normal limits
Distortion product otoacoustic emissions (DPOAE)	Expect reduced amplitude or absent DPOAE at affected frequencies when damage occurs to the outer hair cells.
Auditory evoked potentials	Consistent with audiometric thresholds
Vestibular evaluation	Peripheral findings
Differential diagnosis	Autoimmune inner ear disease, temporal arteritis, Wegener's granulomatosis, Cogan's syndrome, and polyarteritis nodosa, delayed contralateral endolymphatic hydrops, Ménière's disease, acoustic neuroma/ vestibular schwannoma, and ototoxicity (Monsell et al., 2007; National Institute on Deafness and Other Communication Disorders, 2013)

MÉNIÈRE'S DISEASE

Ménière's disease, also known as idiopathic endolymphatic hydrops, is a disorder of the inner ear characterized by four primary symptoms: recurrent episodic vertigo, hearing loss, tinnitus, and aural fullness (American Academy of Otolaryngology-Head and Neck Surgery, 1995). Ménière's disease is a subcategory of the larger Ménière's syndrome, the latter including etiologies such as trauma, viral infection, late stage syphilis, classic or variant Cogan's syndrome, and idiopathic Ménière's disease (Schwaber, 2007). However, Ménière's disease is often used as an umbrella term for all cases of Ménière's syndrome (Schwaber, 2007); therefore, the term Ménière's disease will be used here.

Onset of Ménière's disease typically occurs between the ages of 40 and 60 but it can occur earlier in adulthood (da Costa, de Sousa, & Piza, 2002). Regardless of etiology, the symptoms experienced with Ménière's disease are related to an insufficiency in endolymph absorption (da Costa, de Sousa, & Piza, 2002) and/or volume regulation by the endolymphatic sac, resulting in overaccumulation of endolymph. In turn, the accumulation of fluid displaces membranous structures of the cochlea and/or vestibular organs (Salt & Plontke, 2011), and symptoms result. However, Ménière's disease diagnosis can be challenging because the primary symptoms associated with this disorder are rarely present simultaneously; it might take a year or more for all symptoms to manifest (Schlauch & Nelson, 2015).

Consistent with the variable symptom onset and presentation, Ménière's disease diagnosis can be definite or probable (Committee for an International Classification of Vestibular Disorders, 2015).

Definite Ménière's Disease:

- At least two or more spontaneous episodes of vertigo, each episode lasting 20 minutes to 12 hours
- Low to mid-frequency sensorineural hearing loss with the affected ear at least 30 dB poorer at each of two contiguous frequencies below 2000 Hz. For bilateral cases, the sensory/neural hearing loss should be 35 dB or greater at each of two contiguous frequencies below 2000 Hz.
- Fluctuating aural symptoms (hearing, tinnitus or fullness) in the affected ear; this can manifest on serial audiograms
- Symptoms and findings not better accounted for by another vestibular diagnosis

Probable Ménière's Disease:

- Two or more episodes of vertigo or dizziness, each lasting 20 minutes to 24 hours
- Fluctuating aural symptoms (hearing, tinnitus or fullness) in the reported ear during an episode
- Symptoms and findings not better accounted for by another vestibular diagnosis

When performing pure-tone audiometry on an individual with Ménière's disease, air and bone conduction thresholds should be in agreement and reveal a low-frequency sensorineural hearing loss. In the beginning stages of the disease, hearing sensitivity is normally only affected in one ear, but with time, often progresses to involve both ears (Stahle & Klockhoff, 1986). The results can manifest as a rising configuration, with thresholds increasing by 5 dB or more per octave (Lloyd & Kaplan, 1978). However, perhaps a more common audiometric configuration is one in which mid to high frequencies (at or near 2000 Hz) show 20 dB less hearing loss than lower and higher test frequencies; this configuration is seen in approximately 60% of cases (Schlauch & Nelson, 2015, p. 39).

Early stage Ménière's disease will likely exhibit hearing sensitivity that worsens during episodes of vertigo, but recovers after the attack has ended. In longstanding Ménière's, hearing sensitivity tends to stabilize (Gates, 2006). Ménière's disease is a progressive disorder; however, hearing loss rarely progresses to deafness (Schwaber, 2007).

Y226 tympanograms should be within normal limits. Acoustic reflexes will be normal or at low sensation levels (<60 dBSL) early on due to primarily outer hair cell involvement. Acoustic reflexes may be absent in later stage Ménière's disease (Gates, 2006), reflecting inner hair cell damage. It is likely that distortion product otoacoustic emissions will be reduced or absent in an individual with Ménière's disease; van Huffelen, Mateijesen, and Wit (1998) found them to be present only in approximately 25% of individuals in the early stage of this disorder. ECochG might show an action potential/summating potential amplitude ratio of greater than 0.4. For an overview of expectations see Table 22–7.

Table 22–7. Ménière's Disease

Primary presenting symptom(s)	Sensorineural hearing loss, vertigo, roaring or low pitched tinnitus, and aural fullness or pressure (AAO-HNS, 1995; Lambert, 2000; Committee for an International Classification of Vestibular Disorders, 2015)
Otoscopy	Within normal limits
Weber tuning fork test	Tone is heard at midline for symmetric hearing loss. For asymmetrical hearing losses, if testing at a disordered frequency, tones will be heard in the better ear.
Pure-tone thresholds	Typically a unilateral sensorineural hearing loss, which could progress to bilateral sensorineural hearing loss over time (Stahle & Klockhoff, 1986). Audiometric configurations reported include rising 5 dB or more per octave, or rising 20 dB to a mid-frequency peak at or near 2000 Hz and falling 20 dB or more in the higher test frequencies (Schlauch & Nelson, 2015). See Figure 26-15, Chapter 26.
WRS	Expect good to excellent in early stages, may worsen as the disorder progresses (Gates, 2006).
Y226 Hz tympanometry	Within normal limits
B/G 678 and B/G 1000 Hz tympanometry and middle ear resonance	B/G 678 and B/G 1000 Hz tympanometry within normal limits, resonant frequency might be low but this finding is inconclusive (Franco-Vidal et al., 2005)
G 2000 Hz	Franco-Vidal et al. (2005) suggested 2000 Hz tympanograms are useful in diagnosing active Meniere's disease as conductance (G) will might manifest as width <235 daPa in 95% of normals and >235 daPa in 56.5% of patients with active Ménière's.

Table 22–7. *continued*

Acoustic reflexes	Low sensation level (<60 dB SL) or absent
Wideband acoustic immittance (WAI)	Within normal limits
Distortion product otoacoustic emissions (DPOAE)	Expect reduced or absent DPOAE except early in the disorder's progression when DPOAE is often within normal limits (van Huffelen, Mateijesen, & Wit, 1998).
Auditory evoked potentials	EcochG might show an action potential to summating potential amplitude ratio of greater than 0.4.
Vestibular evaluation	Peripheral findings
Differential diagnosis	Autoimmune inner ear disease, cerebrovascular disease (stroke/TIA), endolymphatic sac tumor, transient ischemic attack, meningiomas, neuroborreliosis, otosyphilis, Susac syndrome, third window syndromes (perilymph fistula, canal dehiscence, enlarged vestibular aqueduct), vestibular migraine, vestibular paroxysmia (neurovascular compression syndrome), vestibular schwannoma, Vogt-Koyanagi-Harada syndrome (Committee for an International Classification of Vestibular Disorders, 2015).

REFERENCES

American Academy of Audiology. (2009*). Position statement and clinical practice guidelines: Ototoxicity monitoring.* Retrieved from http://www.audiology.org/publications-resources/document-library/ototoxicity-monitoring

American Academy of Otolaryngology-Head and Neck Surgery. (1995). Committee on hearing and equilibrium guidelines for the diagnosis and evaluation of therapy in Ménière's disease. *Otolaryngology-Head and Neck Surgery, 113*(3), 181–185.

American Speech-Language-Hearing Association. (1994). *Audiologic management of individuals receiving cochleotoxic drug therapy* [Guidelines]. Retrieved from http://www.asha.org/policy. doi:10.1044/policy.GL1994-00003

Attias J., Ulanovski D. Shemesh, R., Kornreich, L., Nageris, B., Preis, M. . . . Raveh, E. (2012). Air-bone gap component of inner-ear origin in audiograms of cochlear implant candidates. *Otology & Neurotology, 33*, 512–517.

Balkany, T. J., & Dans, P. E. (1978). Reversible sudden deafness in early acquired syphilis. *Archives of Otolaryngology, 104*, 66–68.

Berlow, S. J., Caldarelli, D. D., Matz, G. J., Meyer, D. H., & Harsch, G. G. (1980). Bacterial meningitis and sensorineural hearing loss: A prospective investigation. *Laryngoscope, 90*(9), 1445–1452.

Bilgen, C., Kirkim, G., & Kirazli, T. (2009). Middle ear impedance measurements in large vestibular aqueduct syndrome. *Auris Nasus Larynx, 36*, 263–268.

Campbell A.P., Adunka, O.F., Zhou B, Qaqish, B.F., & Buchman C.A. *(2011).* Large vestibular aqueduct syndrome. *Laryngoscope, 121*, 352–357.

Castellucci, A., Brandolini, C., Piras, G., & Modugno, G. C. (2013). Tympanometric findings in superior semicircular canal dehiscence syndrome. *Acta Otorhinolaryngologica Italica, 33*(2), 112–120. Retrieved from http://www.ncbi.nlm.nih.gov/pmc/articles/PMC3665379/

Chien, W.W., Janky, K., Minor, L.B., & Carey, J.P. (2012). Superior semicircular canal dehiscence size: Multivariate assessment of clinical impact. *Otology and Neurology, 33*, 810–815.

Committee for an International Classification of Vestibular Disorders. (2015). Diagnostic criteria for Menière's disease. *Journal of Vestibular Research, 25*(1), 1–7.

da Costa, S. S., de Sousa, L. C., & Piza, M. R. (2002). Ménière's disease: Overview, epidemiology, and natural history. *Otolaryngologic Clinics of North America, 35*(3), 455–495. http://dx.doi.org/10.1016/S0030-6665(02)00028-2

Dille, M. F., McMillan, G. P., Reavis, K. M., Jacobs, P., Fausti, S. A., & Konrad-Martin, D. (2010). Ototoxicity risk assessment combining distortion product otoacoustic emissions with a cisplatin dose model. *Journal of the Acoustical. Society of America, 128*, 1163–1174. http://dx.doi.org/10.1121/1.3473693

Dobbin, J. M., & Perkins, J. H. (1983). Otosyphilis and hearing loss: Response to penicillin and steroid therapy. *Laryngoscope, 93*(12), 1540–1543.

Fausti, S. A., Henry, J. A., Schaffer, H. I., Olson, D. J., Frey, R. H., & McDonald, W. J. (1992). High frequency audiometric monitoring for early detection of ototoxicity. *Journal of Infectious Disease, 165*, 1026–1032.

Fligor, B., Chasin, M., & Neitzel, R. (2015). Noise exposure. In J. Katz, M. Chasin, K. English, L. Hood, & K. Tillery (Eds.), *Handbook of clinical audiology* (7th ed., pp. 595–616). Philadelphia, PA: Wolters Kluwer.

Franco-Vidal, V., Legarlantezec, C., Blanchet, H., Convert, C., Torti, F., & Darrouzet, V. (2005). Multifrequency admittancemetry in Ménière's disease: A preliminary study for a new diagnostic test. *Otology & Neurology, 26*(4), 723–727.

Gaeth, J. H. (1948). *Study of phonemic regression in relation to hearing loss* [Doctoral dissertation]. Chicago, IL: Northwestern University.

Garcia, V. P., Martinez, F. A., Agusti, E. B., Mencia L. A., & Asenjo, V. P. (2001). Drug induced ototoxicity: Current status. *Acta Otorhinolaryngologica Italica, 121*, 569–572.

Gates, G. A. (2000). Sudden sensorineural hearing loss. In R. F. Canalis & P. R. Lambert (Eds.), *The ear: Comprehensive otology* (pp. 523–536). Philadelphia, PA: Lippincott Williams & Wilkins.

Gates, G. A. (2006). Ménière's disease review 2005. *Journal of the American Academy of Audiology*, *17*, 16–26.

Hanner, P., Rosenhall, U., Edstrom, S., & Kaijser, B. (1989). Hearing impairment in patients with antibody production against Borrelia burgdorferi antigen. *Lancet, 1*, 13–15.

Humes, H. D. (1999). Insights into ototoxicity. Analogies to nephrotoxicity. *Annals of the New York Academy of Sciences*, *884*, 15–18.

Jackler, R. K., & De La Cruz, A. (1989). The large vestibular aqueduct syndrome. *Laryngoscope*, *99*(12), 1238–1243.

Kujawa, S. G., & Liberman, M. C. (2009). Adding insult to injury: Cochlear nerve degeneration after "temporary" noise-induced hearing loss. *Journal of Neuroscience*, *29*(45), 14077–14085.

Lambert, P. R. (2000). History and physical examination of a patient with dizziness. In R. F. Canalis & P. R. Lambert (Eds.), *The ear: Comprehensive otology* (pp. 167–179). Philadelphia, PA: Lippincott Williams & Wilkins.

Levinson, M. J., Parisier, S. C., Jacobs, M., & Edelstein, D. R. (1989). The large vestibular aqueduct syndrome in children: A review of 12 cases and the description of a new clinical entity. *Archives of Otolaryngology*, *115*, 54–58.

Lloyd, L. L., & Kaplan, H. (1978). *Audiometric interpretation: Amanual for basic audiometry.* Baltimore, MD: University Park Press.

Lobarinas, E., Salvi, R., & Ding, D. (2013). Insensitivity of the audiogram to carboplatin-induced inner hair cell loss in chinchillas. *Hearing Research. 302*, 113–120. http://dx.doi.org/10.1016/j.heares.2013.03.012

Lundborg, T. (1980). Clinical experiences with communication instruments in adults with sensorineural hearing loss. *Audiology*, *19*, 189–201.

Mathur, N. N., & Roland, P. S. (2014). *Noise-induced hearing loss differential diagnoses.* Retrieved from http://emedicine.medscape.com/article/857813-differential

McArdle, R., & Hnath-Chisolm, T. (2015). Speech audiometry. In J. Katz, M. Chasin, K. English, L. J. Hood, & K. L. Tillery (Eds.), *Handbook of clinical audiology* (pp. 61–75). Philadelphia, PA: Wolters Kluwer.

Merchant, S. N., Rosowski, J. J., & McKenna, M. J. (2007). Superior semicircular canal dehiscence mimicking otosclerotic hearing loss. *Advances in in Oto-Rhino-Laryngology*, *65*, 137–145.

Mimura, T., Sato, E., Sugiura, M., Yoshino, T., Naganawa, S., & Nakashima, T. (2005). Hearing loss in patients with enlarged vestibular aqueduct: Air-bone gap and audiological Bing test. *International Journal of Audiology*, *44*, 466–469.

Minor, L. B. (2005). Clinical manifestations of superior semicircular canal dehiscence. *Laryngoscope*, *115*, 1717–1727. http://dx.doi.org/10.1097/01.mlg.0000178324.55729.b7

Monsell, E. M., Teixido, M. T., Slattery, E. L., Wilson, M. D., Kung, B., & Hughes, G. B. (2007). Pure-tone evaluation. In G. Hughes & M. Pensak (Eds.), *Clinical otology* (pp. 300–320). New York, NY: Thieme Medical.

Nakajima, H. H., Pisano, D. V., Roosli, C., Hamade, M. A., Merchant, G. R., Mahfood, L., . . . Merchant, S. N. (2012). Comparison of ear-canal reflectance and umbo velocity in patients with conductive hearing loss: A preliminary study. *Ear and Hearing*, *33*(1), 35–43.

National Institute on Deafness and Other Communication Disorders. (2013). *Age-related hearing loss.* Retrieved from http://www.nidcd.nih.gov/health/hearing/Pages/Age-Related-Hearing-Loss.aspx

National Institute on Deafness and Other Communication Disorders. (2013). *Sudden deafness.* Retrieved from http://www.nidcd.nih.gov/health/hearing/pages/sudden.aspx

National Institute on Deafness and Other Communication Disorders. (2014). *Noise-induced hearing loss.* Retrieved from http://www.nidcd.nih.gov/health/hearing/pages/noise.aspx

Paparella, M. M., Morizono, T., Le, C. T., Mancini, F., Sipilä, P., Choo, Y. B., Lidén, G., & Kim, C. S. (1984). Sensorineural hearing loss in otitis media. *Annals of Otology, Rhinology, and Laryngology*, *93*(6 Pt. 1), 623–629.

Peltomaa, M., Pyykkö, I., Seppälä, I., Viitanen, L., & Viljanen, M. (2000). Lyme borreliosis, an etiological factor in sensorineural hearing loss? *European Archives of Oto-Rhino Laryngology*, *257*(6), 317–322.

Rabinowitz, P. M. (2000). Noise-induced hearing loss. *American Family Physician*, *61*(9), 2749–2756.

Roland, P. S. (2015). *Presbycusis.* Retrieved from http://reference.medscape.com/article/855989-overview

Rosowski, J. J., Songer, J. E., Nakajima, H. H., Brinsko, K. M., & Merchant, S. N. (2004). Clinical, experimental, and theoretical investigations of the effect of superior semicircular canal dehiscence on hearing mechanisms. *Otology & Neurotology*, *25*(3), 323–332.

Salt, A. N., & Plontke, S. K. (2011). Endolymphatic hydrops: Pathophysiology and experimental models. *Otolaryngologic Clinics of North America*, *43*(5), 971–983. http://dx.doi.org/10.1016/j.otc.2010.05.007

Sato, E., Nakashima, T., Lilly, D.J., Fausti, S.A., Ueda, H., Misawa, H., & Naganawa, S. (2002). Tympanometric findings in patients with enlarged vestibular aqueducts. *Laryngoscope*, *112*(9), 1642–1646.

Schlauch, R. S., & Nelson, P. (2015). Pure-tone evaluation. In J. Katz, M. Chasin, K. English, L. J. Hood, & K. L. Tillery (Eds.), *Handbook of clinical audiology* (pp. 29–47). Philadelphia, PA: Wolters Kluwer.

Schuknecht, H. F. (1964). Further observations on the pathology of presbycusis. *Archives of Otolaryngology*, *80*(4), 369–382. http://dx.doi.org/10.1001/archotol.1964.00750040381003

Schuknecht, H. F., & Gacek, M. R. (1993). Cochlear pathology in presbycusis. *Annals of Otology, Rhinology, and Laryngology*, *102*(1 Pt 2), 1–16.

Schwaber, M. K. (2007). Vestibular disorders. In G. Hughes & M. Pensak (Eds.), *Clinical otology* (pp. 355–374). New York, NY: Thieme Medical.

Stahle J., & Klockhoff I. (1986). Diagnostic procedures, differential diagnosis, and general conclusions. In C.

R. Pfaltz (Ed.), *Controversial aspects of Ménière disease* (pp. 71–86). New York, NY: Thieme.

Suzuka, Y., & Schuknecht, H. F. (1988). Retrograde cochlear neuronal degeneration in human subjects. *Acta Otolaryngologica Italica, Suppl., 450*, 1–20.

van Huffelen, W., Mateijesen, N., & Wit, H. (1998). Classification of patients with Ménière's disease using otoacoustic emissions. *Audiology and Neurotology, 3*, 419–430.

Weinstein, B. E. (2015). Hearing loss in the elderly: A new look at an old problem. In J. Katz, M. Chasin, K. English, L. Hood, & K. Tillery (Eds.), *Handbook of clinical audiology* (7th ed., pp. 631–645). Philadelphia, PA: Wolters Kluwer.

23

VIII Nerve/Brainstem Disorders

AUDITORY NEUROPATHY SPECTRUM DISORDER

Auditory neuropathy spectrum disorder (ANSD), also known as auditory neuropathy and auditory dys-synchrony, involves disorder at the level of the inner hair cells (Amatuzzi et al., 2001), cranial nerve VIII (Starr, Picton, Sininger, Hood, & Berlin, 1996), and/or brainstem (Berlin, Hood, Morlet, Rose, & Brashears, 2003). Neural involvement might include insufficient myelination of auditory nerve fibers (Starr et al., 2001) or kernicteric deposits due to hyperbilirubinemia (Shapiro & Nakamura, 2001). ANSD can be either congenital or acquired, and approximately 90% of diagnosed cases occur bilaterally (Picton, 2011). Risk factors for ANSD include premature birth, hyperbilirubinemia, anoxia, hypoxia, congenital brain anomalies, ototoxic drug exposure, and genetics (Manchaiah, Zhao, Danesh, & Duprey, 2011).

With ANSD, pure-tone thresholds can range from within normal limits to profound hearing loss (Doyle, Sininger, & Starr, 1998; NIDCD, 2003).

Word recognition scores are typically poorer than expected based on the audiogram. Expect normal OAE results, a finding important to consider during newborn infant hearing screenings.

Y226 tympanometry will be within normal limits. When testing acoustic reflexes at 1000 Hz and 2000 Hz, Berlin et al. (2005) reported at least one of those thresholds were >95 dB HL in his subjects with ANSD. Approximately 75% of patients with ANSD will have no discernable repeatable ABR waves, while the remainder will show low amplitude responses at high intensity levels (Berlin et al., 2001). Cochlear microphonics will, however, be preserved (Starr, Picton, Sininger, Hood, & Berlin, 1996). Responses obtained using high-intensity level condensation clicks might reveal an inverted waveform compared to responses obtained with rarefaction clicks (Berlin et al., 1998). For an overview of expectations see Table 23–1.

Table 23–1. Auditory Neuropathy Spectrum Disorder

Primary presenting symptom(s)	Hearing loss and difficulty understanding speech, especially in the presence of noise (Starr, Picton, Sininger, Hood, & Berlin, 1996).
Otoscopy	Within normal limits
Weber tuning fork test	Tone is heard at midline for symmetric hearing loss. For asymmetrical hearing losses, if testing at a disordered frequency, tones will be heard in the better ear.
Pure-tone thresholds	Variable; results may range from within normal limits to a profound hearing loss (Doyle, Sininger, & Starr, 1998; NIDCD, 2003); air- and bone-conduction thresholds will be similar.

Table 23–1. *continued*

WRS	Poorer WRS than would be expected based on audiometric thresholds (Doyle et al., 1998).
Y226 Hz tympanometry	Within normal limits
B/G 678 and B/G 1000 Hz tympanometry and middle ear resonance	Within normal limits
Acoustic reflex thresholds	Generally >95 dB HL (Berlin, 2005); when testing at 1000 Hz and 2000 Hz, Berlin reported at least one of those acoustic reflex thresholds were >95 dB HL.
Wideband acoustic immittance (WAI)	Within normal limits.
Distortion product otoacoustic emissions (DPOAE)	Present in the initial stages (Starr et al., 1996; Berlin et al., 2005)
Auditory evoked potentials	No discernable repeatable ABR waves or low amplitude responses at high intensity levels (Berlin, Hood, & Rose, 2001). Responses obtained using high intensity level condensation clicks might reveal an inverted waveform compared to responses obtained with rarefaction clicks (Berlin et al., 1998). Cochlear microphonics however, will be preserved (Starr et al., 1996).
Differential diagnosis	Central auditory processing disorder, acoustic neuroma/vestibular schwannoma

VESTIBULAR SCHWANNOMA

Vestibular schwannomas, also referred to as acoustic neuromas, are typically benign and slow-growing neoplasms of CN VIII (Feeney & Schairer, 2015) at the rate of 0.15 to 0.2 cm in diameter annually (Bederson, von Ammon, Wichmann, & Yasargil, 1991). The vast majority of vestibular schwannomas are unilateral, with bilateral cases occurring primarily in individuals with neurofibromatosis type 2 (Mayo Clinic, 2014). Eckermeier, Pirsig, and Mueller (1979) found that approximately one-third of cases of vestibular schwannoma in their study displayed CN VII involvement, and other cranial nerves and the brainstem can be affected (Eidelman, 1987). Vestibular schwannomas are the most common mass in the cerebellopontine angle, accounting for 90% of all tumors located in this region (Brackmann & Bartels, 1980). Neoplasms such as meningioma, facial, schwannoma/neuroma, and hemangioma may also affect CN VIII, and produce similar symptoms as vestibular schwannoma (Lustig & Jackler, 2007).

The term vestibular schwannoma is preferred over acoustic neuroma because most of these neoplasms originate in the vestibular branch of CN VIII (Sterkers, Perre, Viala, & Foncin, 1987), specifically from the Schwann cells. Vestibular schwannomas typically must compromise auditory neurons and cause hearing loss in order to be detected; that is, when the tumor has reached 1 to 4 cm (Hall, 1992). Vestibular symptoms are not widely experienced, likely because the slow-growing nature of vestibular schwannomas allows compensation by higher order processes (Hall, 1992).

Asymmetric symptoms and audiometrics are important indicators; see Chapter 27 for discussion and criteria. Hearing loss from vestibular schwannomas is typically sensory/neural with air- and bone-conduction thresholds in agreement. The hearing loss typically begins in higher test frequencies because neurons innervating the base of the cochlea are found on the outer-most portion of CN VIII, and are thus affected by neoplasms in the internal auditory meatus (Schlauch, Levine, Li, & Haines, 1995). Compression of blood vessels in the internal auditory meatus can also cause damage to the auditory nerve and cochlea (Suga & Lindsay, 1976), suggesting mechanism for sudden onset of hearing loss that occurs in an estimated 25% of individuals with vestibular schwannoma (Selesnick, Jackler, & Pitts, 1993).

Y226 tympanometry will be within normal limits, but acoustic reflexes will be absent when stimulating an affected VIII nerve or measuring on the side of an affected VII nerve. DPOAE will be reduced amplitude or absent when blood flow is compromised and outer hair cells are damaged. ABR waves on the affected side will show long latencies and/or abnormal morphology. For an overview of expectations see Table 23–2.

Table 23–2. Vestibular Schwannoma

Primary presenting symptom(s)	Expect unilateral hearing loss with difficulty understanding in the affected ear (Hall, 1992). Onset is typically gradual, but sudden hearing loss is possible (Selesnick et al., 1993). Other symptoms might include unilateral or asymmetric tinnitus, dizziness, unsteadiness, and facial numbness or weakness (Mayo Clinic, 2014).
Otoscopy	Within normal limits
Weber tuning fork test	Tone is heard at midline for symmetric hearing loss. For asymmetrical hearing losses, if testing at a disordered frequency, tones will be heard in the better ear.
Pure-tone thresholds	Results are variable; results may range from within normal limits to profound sensorineural hearing loss. Due to the tonotopic organization of the auditory nerve, high frequencies are typically affected first (Schlauch et al., 1995). See Figure 26–16 in Chapter 26.
WRS	Poorer than would be expected in the affected ear.
Y226 Hz tympanometry	Within normal limits
Resonant peak and B/G 678 Hz tympanometry	Within normal limits
Acoustic reflexes	Elevated or absent when stimulating an affected VIII nerve (Jerger, Harford, Clemis, & Alford, 1974) or measuring on the side of an affected VII nerve
Wideband acoustic immittance (WAI)	Within normal limits

Table 23–2. *continued*

Distortion product otoacoustic emissions (DPOAE)	Reduced or absent when outer hair cells are damaged by reduced blood flow
Auditory evoked potentials	ABR waves on the affected side will show long latencies and/or abnormal morphology.
Vestibular evaluation	Peripheral findings
Differential diagnosis	Sudden idiopathic sensory/neural hearing loss, presbyacusis, noise-induced hearing loss

REFERENCES

Amatuzzi, M. G., Northrop, C., Liberman, M. C., Thornton, A., Halpin, C., Herrmann, B., . . . Eavey, R. D. (2001). Selective inner hair cell loss in premature infants and cochlea pathological patterns from neonatal intensive care unit autopsies. *Archives of Otolaryngology-Head and Neck Surgery*, *127*, 629–636.

Bederson, J. B., von Ammon, K., Wichmann, W. W., & Yasargil, M. G. (1991). Conservative treatment of patients with acoustic tumors. *Neurosurgery*, *28*(5), 646-650.

Berlin, C. I., Bordelon, J., St. John, P., Wilensky, D., Hurley, A., Kluka, E., & Hood, L. J. (1998). Reversing click polarity may uncover auditory neuropathy in infants. *Ear and Hearing*, *19*(1), 37–47.

Berlin, C. I., Hood, L. J., Morlet, T., Rose, K., & Brashears, S. (2003). Auditory neuropathy/dys-synchrony: Diagnosis and management. *Mental Retardation And Developmental Disabilities Research Reviews*, *9*, 225–231.

Berlin, C. I., Hood, L. J., Morlet, T., Wilensky, D., St. John, P., Montgomery, E., & Thibodaux, M. (2005). Absent or elevated middle ear muscle reflexes in the presence of normal otoacoustic emissions: A universal finding in 136 cases of auditory neuropathy/dys-synchrony. *Journal of the American Academy of Audiology, 16*(8), 546–553.

Berlin, C. I., Hood, L. J., & Rose, K. (2001). On renaming auditory neuropathy as auditory dys-synchrony: Implications for a clearer understanding of the underlying mechanisms and management options. *Audiology Today, 13*(6), 15–17.

Brackmann, D. E., & Bartels, L. J. (1980). Rare tumors of the cerebellopontine angle. *Otolaryngology-Head and Neck Surgery, 88*(5), 555–559.

Doyle, K. J., Sininger, Y. S., & Starr, A. (1998). Auditory neuropathy in children. *Laryngoscope, 108*(9), 1374–1377.

Eckermeier, L., Pirsig, W., & Mueller, D. (1979). Histopathology of 30 non-operated acoustic schwannomas. *Archives of Oto-Rhino-Laryngology, 222*(1), 1–9.

Eidelman, B. H. (1987). Clinical syndromes of the posterior fossa. In L. N. Sekhar & V. L. Schramm (Eds.), *Tumors of the cranial base: Diagnosis and treatment* (pp. 541–543). Mount Kisco, NY: Futura.

Feeney, M. P., & Schairer, K. S. (2015). Acoustic stapedius reflex measurements. In J. Katz, M. Chasin, K. English, L. J. Hood, & K. L. Tillery (Eds.), *Handbook of clinical audiology* (pp. 165-186). Philadelphia, PA: Wolters Kluwer.

Hall, J. W. (1992). *Handbook of auditory evoked potentials*. Boston, MA: Allyn & Bacon.

Jerger, J., Harford, E., Clemis, J., & Alford, B. (1974). The acoustic reflex in eighth nerve disorders. *Archives of Otolaryngology, 99*, 409–413.

Lustig, L. R., & Jackler, R. K. (2007). Benign neoplasms of the temporal bone. In G. B. Hughes & M. L. Pensak (Eds.), *Clinical otology* (pp. 321–338). New York, NY: Thieme Medical.

Manchaiah, V. K., Zhao, F., Danesh, A. A., & Duprey, R. (2011). The genetic basis of auditory neuropathy spectrum disorder (ANSD). *International Journal of Pediatric Otorhinolaryngology*, *75*(2), 151–158. http://dx.doi.org/10.1016/j.ijporl.2010.11.023

Mayo Clinic. (2014). *Acoustic neuroma.* Retrieved from http://www.mayoclinic.org/diseases-conditions/acoustic-neuroma/basics/treatment/con-20023851

National Institute on Deafness and Other Communication Disorders. (2003). *Auditory neuropathy.* Retrieved from http://www.nidcd.nih.gov/health/hearing/pages/neuropathy.aspx

Picton, T. W. (2011). *Human auditory-evoked potentials.* San Diego: Plural.

Schlauch, R. S., Levine, S., Li, Y., & Haines, S. (1995). Evaluating hearing threshold differences between ears as a screen for acoustic neuroma. *Journal of Speech and Hearing Research*, *38*, 1168–1175.

Selesnick, S. H., Jackler, R. K., & Pitts, L. W. (1993). The changing clinical presentation of acoustic tumors in the MRI era. *Laryngoscope*, *103*(4), 431–436.

Shapiro, S. M,. & Nakamura, H. (2001). Bilirubin and the auditory system. *Journal of Perinatology*, *21*(8), S52–S55.

Starr, A., Picton, T. W., & Kim, R. (2001). Pathophysiology of auditory neuropathy. In Y. S. Sininger & A. Starr (Eds.), *Auditory neuropathy: A new perspective on hearing disorders* (pp. 67–82). San Diego, CA: Singular Thomson Learning.

Starr, A., Picton, T. W., Sininger, Y., Hood, L. J., & Berlin, C. I. (1996). Auditory neuropathy. *Brain*, *139*(2), 741–753.

Sterkers, J. M., Perre, J., Viala, P., & Foncin, J. F. (1987). The origin of acoustic neuromas. *Acta Otolaryngologica*, *103*(5–6), 427–431.

Suga, F., & Lindsay, J. R. (1976). Inner ear degeneration in acoustic neurinoma. *Annals of Otology, Rhinology & Laryngology*, *85*(3), 343–358. http://dx.doi.org/10.1177/000348947608500305

24

Systemic Disorders

DIABETES MELLITUS

Diabetes mellitus is a disease in which blood glucose levels exceed that of a non-diabetic individual (National Institute of Diabetes and Digestive and Kidney Diseases, 2014). Diabetes mellitus can be divided into a multitude of categories, but two classifications represent chronic diagnoses: Type 1, or insulin-dependent diabetes, and Type 2, or noninsulin-dependent diabetes. Type 1 diabetes occurs when the immune system targets and destroys pancreatic cells in the body that produce insulin, which is the hormone responsible for transporting glucose from the bloodstream to cells of the body for energy use (American Diabetes Association, 2015). High blood glucose levels over time can cause blood vessel and nerve damage leading to a number of further complications (National Institute of Diabetes and Digestive and Kidney Diseases, 2014). There is no cure for Type 1 diabetes, and individuals with this disorder require insulin delivered via injection in order to regulate blood glucose levels (Centers for Disease Control and Prevention,

2011). Type 1 diabetes is much less common than Type 2, accounting for only 5% of all cases, with onset normally during childhood or young adulthood (American Diabetes Association, 2015).

Type 2 diabetes develops when cells begin to resist insulin, causing the pancreas to increase production of this hormone (American Diabetes Association, 2015). Eventually the pancreas might no longer be able to keep up with the demand for insulin, and cells of the body will become energy deficient. Individuals with Type 2 diabetes may be able to regulate blood glucose levels through diet and regular exercise, but otherwise may need to supplement with oral medications or insulin treatments (Mayo Clinic, 2014). Risk factors for developing Type 2 diabetes include "older age, obesity, family history of diabetes, history of gestational diabetes, impaired glucose metabolism, and physical inactivity" (CDC, 2011, p. 11).

Researchers have found an association between diabetes and hearing loss; elevated blood glucose levels could cause blood vessel damage within the cochlea. Among diabetics there is a greater prevalence of low-frequency to mid-frequency hearing loss, and also a higher prevalence of high-frequency hearing impairment (Bainbridge, Hoffman & Cowie, 2008).

Expect sensorineural hearing loss, air conduction and bone thresholds will be in agreement, except in rare cases when concomitant malignant otitis adds a conductive component due to vulnerability of infection and inability to heal that occurs with diabetes (Casqueiro, Casqueiro, & Alves, 2012). Y226 Hz tympanograms will be within normal limits. Acoustic reflex thresholds will likely be measured at low sensation levels (<60 dB SL) when stimulating an ear with mild to moderate cochlear loss, the greater the hearing loss the more likely acoustic reflex thresholds will be elevated or absent due to inner hair cell damage. Distortion product otoacoustic emission amplitudes will be reduced or absent, depending on the degree of hearing loss and at frequencies at which hearing loss is present. Due to auditory neuropathy (Rance et al., 2014), patients with diabetes might have slightly longer ABR wave V latencies (Konrad-Martin et al., 2010). For an overview of expectations see Table 24–1.

CARDIOVASCULAR DISORDER

Cardiovascular disease (CVD) is an inclusive term referring to dysfunction of the heart or blood vessels (American Heart Association, 2014). Resulting impairments of blood supply to sensory/neural structures have been associated with sensory/neural hearing loss (Hull & Kerschen, 2010), for example, by a narrowing of the internal auditory artery (Brant et al., 1996; Fisch, Bobozi, & Greig, 1972; Makishima, 1978). Associated hearing loss risk factors include smoking, noise exposure, and cardiorespiratory fitness (Hutchinson & Alessio, 2010).

Rubinstein, Hildesheimer, Zohar & Chilarovitz, (1997) found a significant difference in the puretone thresholds of older adults with CVD when compared to older adults without CVD. This could be due to degeneration of the stria vascularis disrupting the production of endolymph (Graton, Schmiedt, & Schulte, 1996; Schuknecht & Gacek, 1993). Friedland, Cederberg, and Tarima (2009) recommended that patients be evaluated for CVD if they present with presbycusis and flat or gently sloping strial audiogram configurations. By extension, we recommend that physicians refer any CVD patients for an audiologic evaluation.

Table 24–1. Diabetes Mellitus

Primary presenting symptom(s)	Gradual hearing loss with history of diabetes
Otoscopy	Within normal limits
Weber tuning fork test	Tone is heard at midline for symmetric hearing loss. For asymmetrical hearing losses, if testing at a disordered frequency, tones will be heard in the better ear.
Pure-tone thresholds	Sensorineural low, mid and/or high-frequency hearing loss (Figure 26–17, Chapter 26)
WRS	Good unless inner hair cells and/or neurons are damaged, the greater the inner hair cell damage, the poorer the WRS (McArdle & Hnath-Chisolm, 2015); neural involvement typically will not affect WRS in quiet
Y226 Hz tympanometry	Within normal limits
B/G 678 and B/G 1000 Hz tympanometry and middle ear resonance	Within normal limits
Acoustic reflex thresholds	Present at low sensation levels with outer hair cell damage only, elevated or absent when inner hair cells are damaged
Wideband acoustic immittance (WAI)	Within normal limits
Distortion product otoacoustic emissions (DPOAE)	Reduced amplitude or absent depending on the degree of hearing loss and outer hair cell damage at frequencies where there is hearing loss

Table 24–1. *continued*

Auditory evoked potentials	Slightly delayed wave V latencies
Vestibular evaluation	This may reveal peripheral (VIII nerve) or central (brainstem) findings, especially with patients who have experienced a longer duration of disease. Vestibular dysfunction is considered to be separate and unrelated to neural damage of the eyes and limbs that occurs with this disease (Agrawal et al., 2010).
Differential diagnosis	Children (under the age of 25): Wolfram syndrome, Alstrom syndrome, Wolcott-Rallison syndrome, and Maturity-onset diabetes of the young (Barrent, 2007)
	Adults: Presbycusis, noise-induced hearing loss, cardiovascular disease

Pure-tone audiometry air- and bone-conduction thresholds should be in agreement and may reveal flat or gently sloping strial audiogram configurations (Gates, Cobb, D'Agostino, & Wolf, 1993; Friedland et al., 2009). Y226 tympanometry results will be within normal limits. Acoustic reflexes will likely be measured at low sensation levels (<60 dB SL) at frequencies in which largely outer hair cell disorder has occurred. When inner hair cells are involved, acoustic reflexes will be elevated or absent. Similarly, OAE's will likely be reduced or absent at frequencies in which there is outer hair cell disorder. For an overview of expectations see Table 24–2.

Table 24–2. Cardiovascular Disorder

Primary presenting symptom(s)	Progressive hearing loss of gradual onset
Otoscopy	Normal
Weber tuning fork test	Tone is heard at midline for symmetric hearing loss. For asymmetrical hearing losses, if testing at a disordered frequency, tones will be heard in the better ear.
Pure-tone thresholds	Variable; flat or gently sloping sensorineural hearing loss has been reported in cases of restricted blood supply to the cochlea (Gates et al., 1993; Friedland et al., 2009) while increased blood pressure has been associated with mid-high frequency hearing loss (Brant et al., 1996) (Figure 26–17, Chapter 26).
WRS	Good unless inner hair cells are damaged, the greater the inner hair cell damage the poorer the WRS (McArdle & Hnath-Chisolm, 2015)
Y226 Hz tympanometry	Within normal limits
B/G 678 and B/G 1000 Hz tympanometry and middle ear resonance	Within normal limits
Acoustic reflexes	Low sensation level with outer hair cell disorder only, elevated or absent when inner hair cells are disordered
Wideband acoustic immittance (WAI)	Within normal limits

Table 24–2. *continued*

Distortion product otoacoustic emissions (DPOAE)	Reduced amplitude or absent reflecting outer hair cell disorder
Auditory evoked potentials	Consistent with audiometric thresholds
Differential diagnosis	Presbyacusis and comorbidity with diabetes

REFERENCES

Agrawal, Y., Carey, J., Della Santina, C., Schubert, M., & Minor, L. (2010). Diabetes, vestibular dysfunction, and falls: Analyses from the National Health and Nutrition Examination Survey. *Otology & Neurology, 31(9)*, 1445–1450.

American Diabetes Association. (2015). *Diabetes basics.* Retrieved from http://www.diabetes.org/diabetes-basics/type-1/

American Heart Association. (2014). *What is cardiovascular disease?* Retrieved from http://www.heart.org/HEARTORG/Caregiver/Resources/WhatisCardiovascularDisease/What-is-Cardiovascular-Disease_UCM_301852_Article.jsp#.Vx96yU32bcs

Atcherson, S. R., & Stoody, T. M. (2012). *Auditory electrophysiology: A clinical guide.* New York, NY: Thieme Medical.

Bainbridge, K. E., Hoffman, H. J., & Cowie, C. C. (2008). Diabetes and hearing impairment in the United States: Audiometric evidence from the National Health and

Nutrition Examination Survey, 1999 to 2004. *Annals of Internal Medicine*, *149*(1), 1–10.

Barrent, T. G. (2007). Differential diagnosis of type 1 diabetes: Which genetic syndromes need to be considered? *Pediatric Diabetes*, *8*, 15–23. Retrieved from http://onlinelibrary.wiley.com/doi/10.1111/j.1399-5448.2007.00278.x/full

Brant, L. J., Gordon-Salant, S., Pearson, J. D., Klein, L. L., Morrell, C. H., & Metter, E. J. (1996). Risk factors related to age-associated hearing loss in the speech frequencies. *Journal of the American Academy of Audiology*, *7*, 152–160.

Casqueiro, J., Casqueiro, J., & Alves, C. (2012). Infections in patients with diabetes mellitus: A review of pathogenesis. *Indian Journal of Endocrinology and Metabolism*, *16*, 27–36. http://dx.doi.org/10.4103/2230-8210.94253

Centers for Disease Control and Prevention. (2011). *National diabetes fact sheet: National estimates and general information on diabetes and prediabetes in the United States*. Retrieved from http://www.cdc.gov/diabetes/pubs/pdf/ndfs_2011.pdf

Fisch, U., Bobozi, M., & Greig, D. (1972). Degenerative changes of the arterial vessels of the internal auditory meatus during the process of aging. *Acta Otolaryngologica Italica*, *73*, 259–266.

Friedland, D. R., Cederberg, C., & Tarima, S. (2009). Audiometric pattern as a predictor of cardiovascular status: Development of a model for assessment of risk. *Laryngoscope*, *119*, 473–486.

Gates, G. A. (2000). Sudden sensorineural hearing loss. In R. F. Canalis, & P. R. Lambert (Eds.), *The ear: Comprehensive otology* (pp. 523–536). Philadelphia, PA: Lippincott Williams & Wilkins.

Gates, G. A., Cobb, J. L., D'Agostino, R. B., & Wolf, P. A. (1993). The relation of hearing in the elderly to the presence of cardiovascular disease and cardiovascular risk factors. *Archives of Otolaryngology-Head and Neck Surgery*, *115*, 1227–1230.

Graton, M. A., Schmiedt, R. A., & Schulte, B. A. (1996). Age-related decreases in endocochlear potential are asso-

ciated with vascular abnormalities. *Hearing Research, 94*, 116–124.
Hull, R. H., & Kerschen, S. R. (2010). The influence of cardiovascular health on peripheral and central auditory function in adults: A research review. *American Journal of Audiology, 19*, 9–16. http://dx.doi.org/10.1044/1059-0889(2010/08-0040)
Hutchinson, K. M., & Alessio, H. (2010). Association between cardiovascular health and hearing function: Pure-tone and distortion product otoacoustic emission measures. *American Journal of Audiology, 19*, 26–35. http://dx.doi.org/10.1044/1059-0889(2009/09-0009)
Konrad-Martin, D., Austin, D. F., Griest, S., McMillan, G. P., McDermott, D., & Fausti, S. (2010). Diabetes-related changes in auditory brainstem responses. *Laryngoscope, 120*(1), 150–158.
Makishima, K. (1978). Arteriolar sclerosis as a cause of presbycusis. *Otolaryngology, 86*, 322–326.
Mayo Clinic. (2014.) *Diabetes*. Retrieved from http://www.mayoclinic.org/diseases-conditions/diabetes/basics/tests-diagnosis/con-20033091
Mayo Clinic. (2014). *Heart disease*. Retrieved from http://www.mayoclinic.org/diseases-conditions/heart-disease/basics/symptoms/CON-20034056
McArdle, R., & Hnath-Chisolm, T. (2015). Speech audiometry. In J. Katz, M. Chasin, K. English, L. Hood, & K. Tillery (Eds.), *Handbook of clinical audiology* (7th ed., pp. 61–75). Philadelphia, PA: Wolters Kluwer.
National Institute of Diabetes and Digestive and Kidney Diseases. (2014). *Causes of diabetes*. Retrieved from http://www.niddk.nih.gov/health-information/health-topics/Diabetes/causes-diabetes/Pages/index.aspx
Rance, G., Chisari, D., O'Hare, F., Roberts, L., Shaw, J., Jandeleit-Dahm, K., & Szmulewicz, D. (2014). Auditory neuropathy in individuals with type 1 diabetes. *Journal of Neurology, 261*(8), 1531–1536.
Rubenstein, M., Hildesheimer, M., Zohar, S., & Chilarovitz, T. (1997). Chronic cardiovascular pathology and hearing loss in the aged. *Gerontology, 23*, 4–9.

Schlauch, R. S., & Nelson, P. (2015). Pure-tone evaluation. In J. Katz, M. Chasin, K. English, L. Hood, & K. Tillery (Eds.), *Handbook of clinical audiology* (7th ed., pp. 29–47). Philadelphia, PA: Wolters Kluwer.

Schuknecht, H. F., & Gacek, M. R. (1993). Cochlear pathology in presbycusis. *Annals of Otology, Rhinology and Laryngology. 102*(1 Pt. 2), 1–16.

25

Skull Content Disorder: Intracranial Hypertension

INTRACRANIAL HYPERTENSION

Intracranial hypertension with abnormal cerebrospinal fluid flow has been associated with several neurologic conditions, including syrngohydromyelia, Chiari malformations, trauma, tumors, arachnoiditis, subarachnoid hemorrhages, meningitis, and multiple sclerosis (Steiger, Saccone, & Watson, 2007). Clinical manifestations include whooshing pulsatile tinnitus and low-frequency pseudo-sensory/neural hearing loss. The whooshing pulsatile tinnitus might be the result of blood flow arising from circle of Willis or the walls of the dural sinuses (Rudnick & Sismanis, 2005). The sound waves travel through skull fluids and membranes and through the cochlear or vestibular aqueducts to the cochlea (Marchbanks, Burge, Martin, Bateman, Pickard, & Brightwell, 1990). The hearing loss is considered pseudo-sensory/neural because it is not caused by hair cell or neuronal damage. Instead, the hearing loss has been attributed to masking from the pulsatile tinnitus (Rudnick & Sismanis, 2005; Steiger et al., 2007), or elevated fluid pressure stiffening the basilar, oval, and round window membranes and, thus, hindering traveling waves for both air- and, bone-conduction testing (Sismanis, 1987).

When stimulating an affected ear, expect air-conduction and bone-conduction thresholds to be reduced compared to normal as described above. Limited data are available for tympanometry; Steiger et al., 2007 showed increased Y226 Hz admittance and lower resonant frequency in an affected ear. For an overview of expectations see Table 25–1.

Table 25–1. Intracranial Hypertension

Primary presenting symptom(s)	Hearing loss and whooshing pulsatile tinnitus, possible neurologic symptoms included headache, neck pain, visual abnormalities
Otoscopy	Normal
Weber tuning fork test	Tone is heard at midline for symmetric hearing loss. For asymmetrical hearing losses, if testing at a disordered frequency, tones will be heard in the better ear.
Pure-tone thresholds	Pseudo-sensory/neural (Figure 26–18, Chapter 26)
WRS	Good to excellent
Y226 Hz tympanometry	Minimal data available, admittance might be high (Reid et al.,1989; Marchbanks, Reid, Martin, Brightwell, & Bateman 1987; Steiger et al., 2007)
B/G 678 and B/G 1000 Hz tympanometry and middle ear resonance	Minimal data available, resonance might be lowered (Steiger et al., 2007)
Acoustic reflex thresholds	Variable depending on degree of hearing loss (Reid et al., 1989)
Wideband acoustic immittance (WAI)	No data available
Distortion product otoacoustic emissions (DPOAE)	Variable depending on degree of hearing loss
Auditory evoked potentials	Prolonged wave V latency (Moss, Fino, Patel, & Stone, 2014).

continues

Table 25–1. *continued*

Vestibular evaluation	Low VEMP thresholds on the affected side (Minor, 2005)
Differential diagnosis	Ménière's disease, third-window disorders

REFERENCES

Marchbanks, R. A., Burge, D. M., Martin, A. M., Bateman, D. E., Pickard, J., & Brightwell, A. P. (1990). The relationship between intracranial pressure and tympanic membrane displacement. *British Journal of Audiology, 24*(2), 123–129.

Marchbanks, R. J., Reid, A., Martin, A. M., Brightwell, A. P., & Bateman, D. (1987). The effect of raised intracranial pressure on intracochlear fluid pressure: Three case studies. *British Journal of Audiology 21*(2). http://dx.doi.org/10.3109/03005368709077785

Minor, L. B. (2005). Clinical manifestations of superior semicircular canal dehiscence. *Laryngoscope, 115*, 1717–1727. http://dx.doi.org/10.1097/01.mlg.0000178324.55729.b7

Moss, H., Fino, J., Patel, H., & Stone, J. (2014). Modified brainstem auditory evoked responses are associated with elevated intracranial pressure in subjects with idiopathic intracranial hypertension. *Neurology, 82*(10), 282. Retrieved from http://www.neurology.org/content/82/10_Supplement/P2.282.short

Reid, A., Marchabanks, R. J., Bateman, D. E., Martin, A. M., Brightwell, A. P., & Pickard, J. D. (1989). Mean intracranial pressure monitoring by a non-invasive audiological technique: A pilot study. *Journal of Neurology, Neurosurgery & Psychiatry, 52*, 610–612. http://dx.doi.org/10.1136/jnnp.52.5.610

Rudnick, E., & Sismanis, A. (2005). Pulsatile tinnitus and spontaneous cerebrospinal fluid rhinorrhea: Indicators of benign intracranial hypertension syndrome. *Otology & Neurotology*, *26*(2), 166–168.

Sismanis A. (1987). Otologic manifestations of benign intracranial hypertension syndrome. *Laryngoscope*, *97*(8, Pt. 2, Suppl. 42), 1–17.

Steiger, J.R., Saccone, P., & Watson K.N. (2007). Assessment of objective pulsatile tinnitus in a patient with syringohydromyelia. *Journal of the American Academy of Audiology*, *18*(3), 197–206.

26

Select Audiogram Examples

Of course, the degree of hearing loss of any pathology can vary for many reasons, including the type and degree of disorder and patient characteristics such as age and general health. Moreover, disorders don't always occur in isolation; for example someone with presbyacusis can develop otitis media. Nonetheless, we have included some select audiogram examples to illustrate a possible audiometric configuration for each of several select disorders.

MIDDLE EAR

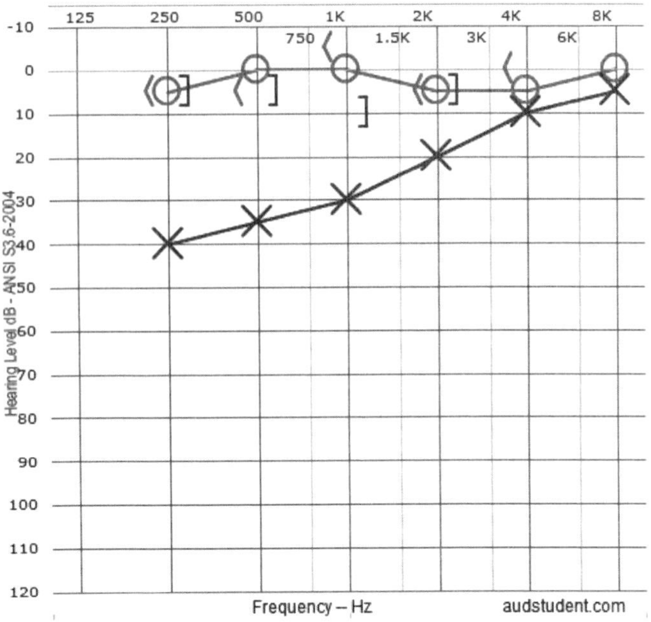

Figure 26–1. Example audiogram for left ear otitis media.

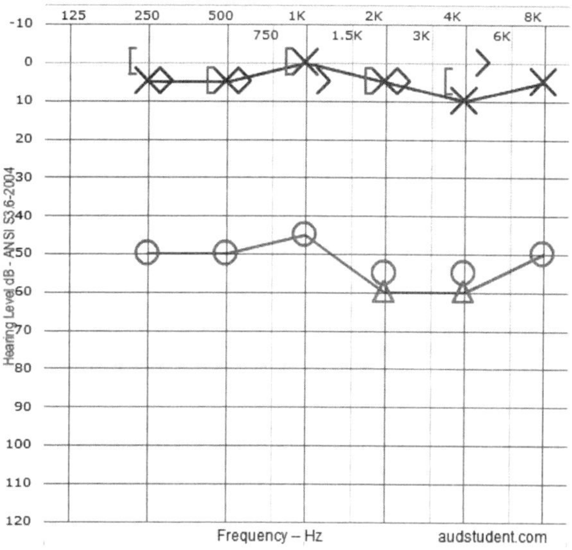

Figure 26–2. Example audiogram for right ear ossicular discontinuity.

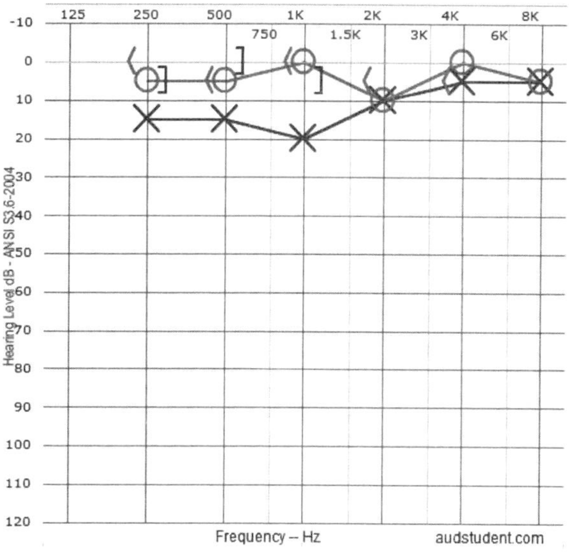

Figure 26–3. Example audiogram for a left glomus tumor.

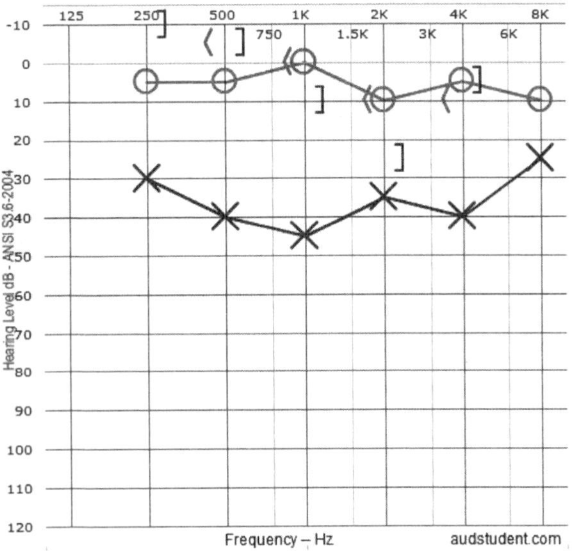

Figure 26–4. Example audiogram for left ossicular fixation due to otosclerosis.

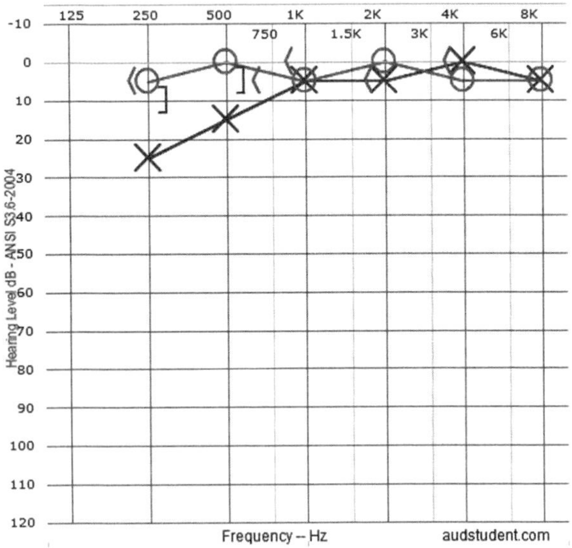

Figure 26–5. Example audiogram for a left tympanic membrane perforation.

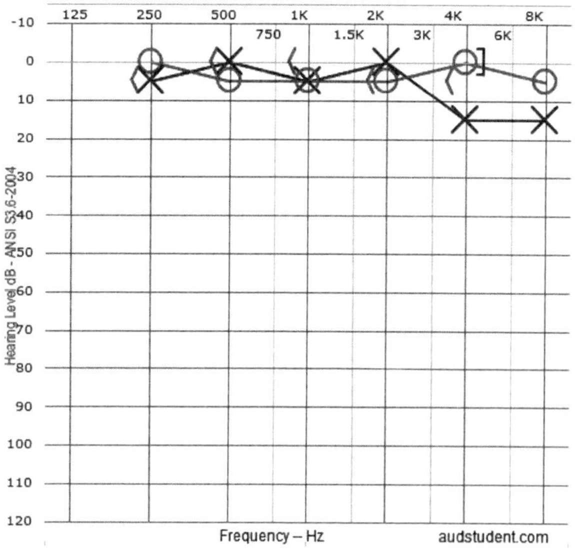

Figure 26–6. Example audiogram for a left monomer/dimer.

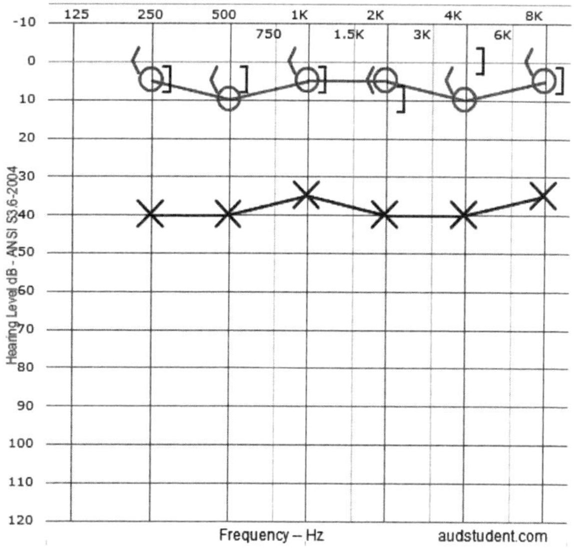

Figure 26–7. Example audiogram for a left ear cholesteatoma.

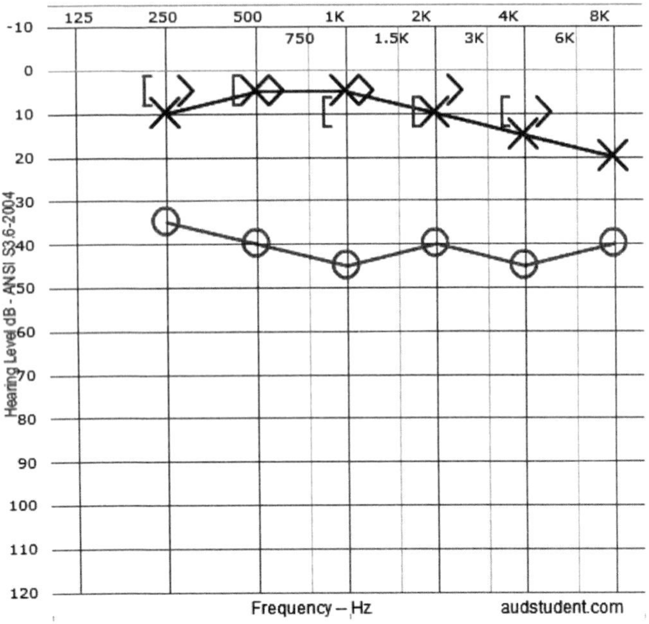

Figure 26–8. Example audiogram for a right cerumen occlusion.

INNER EAR

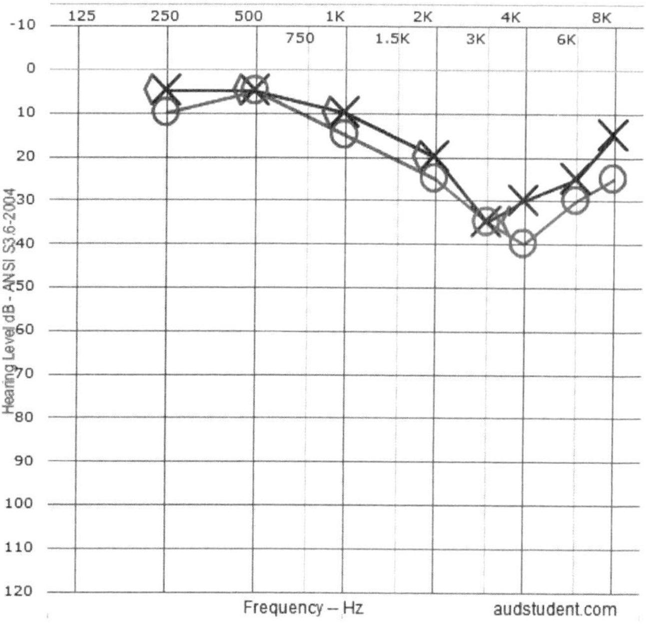

Figure 26–9. Example audiogram for bilateral noise-induced hearing loss.

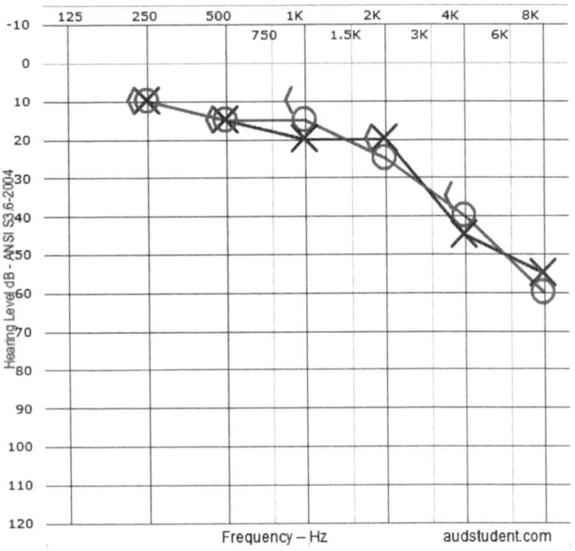

Figure 26–10. Example audiogram for bilateral presbycusis.

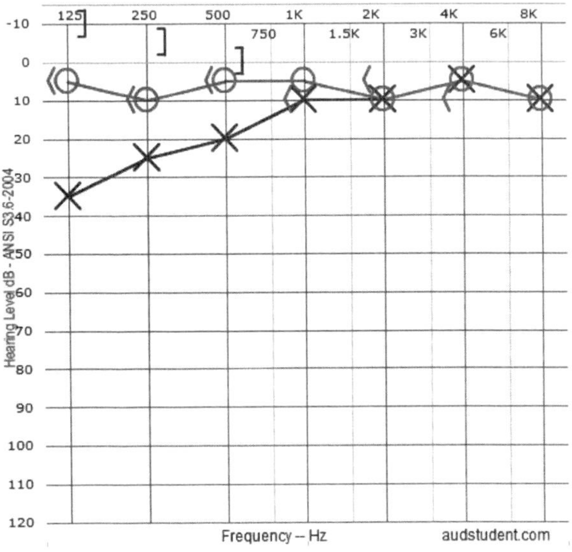

Figure 26–11. Example audiogram for left superior semicircular canal dehiscence.

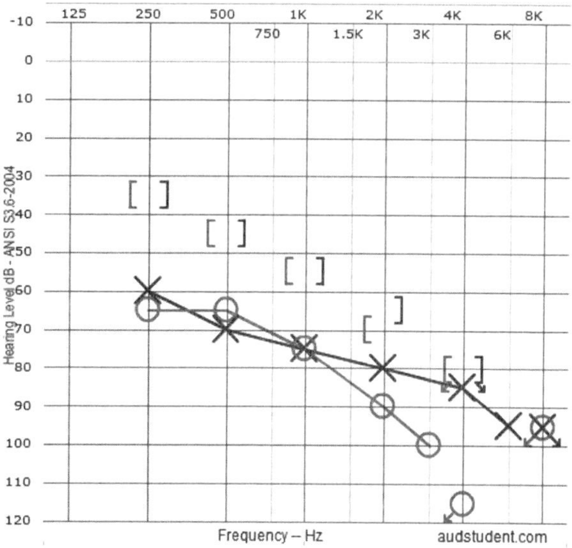

Figure 26–12. Example audiogram for bilateral large vestibular aqueducts.

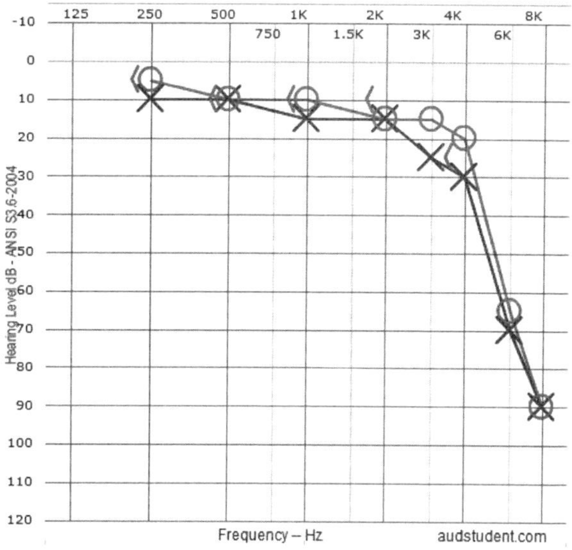

Figure 26–13. Example audiogram for bilateral ototoxicity.

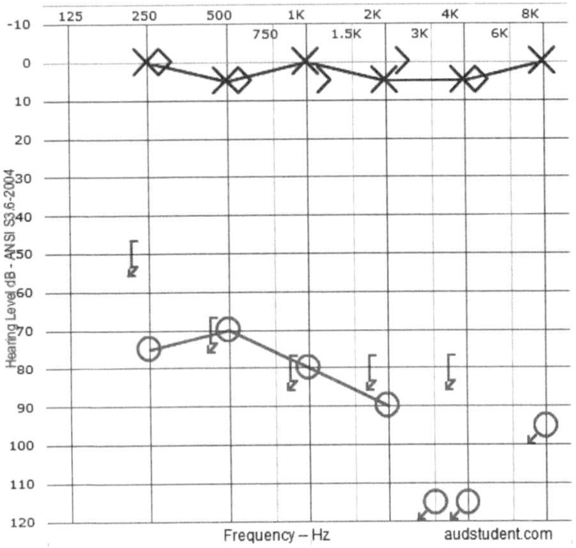

Figure 26–14. Example audiogram for right inner ear infection.

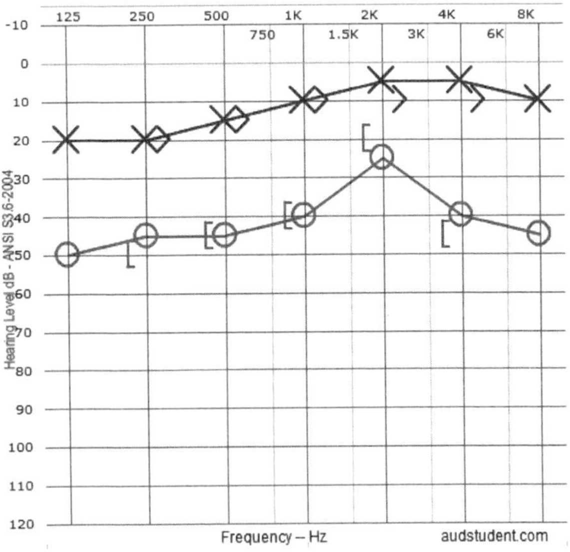

Figure 26–15. Example audiogram for Ménière's disease affecting the right ear more than the left.

VIII NERVE/BRAINSTEM

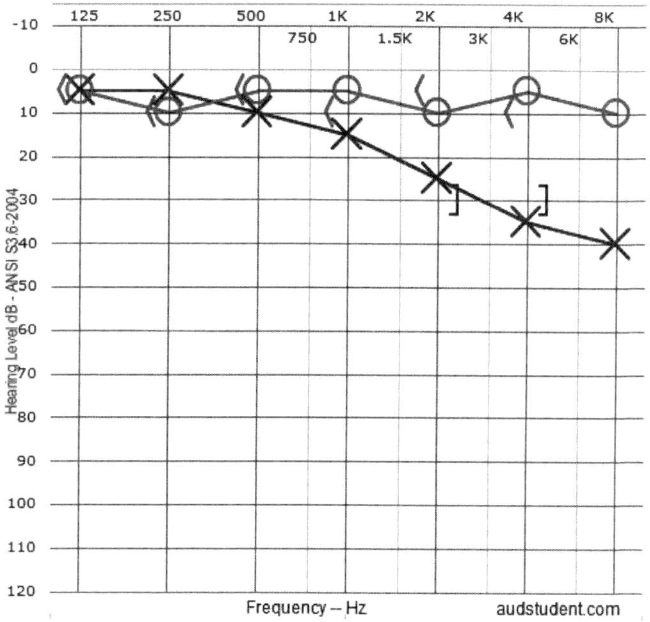

Figure 26–16. Example audiogram for left VIII nerve vestibular schwannoma.

SYSTEMIC DISORDERS

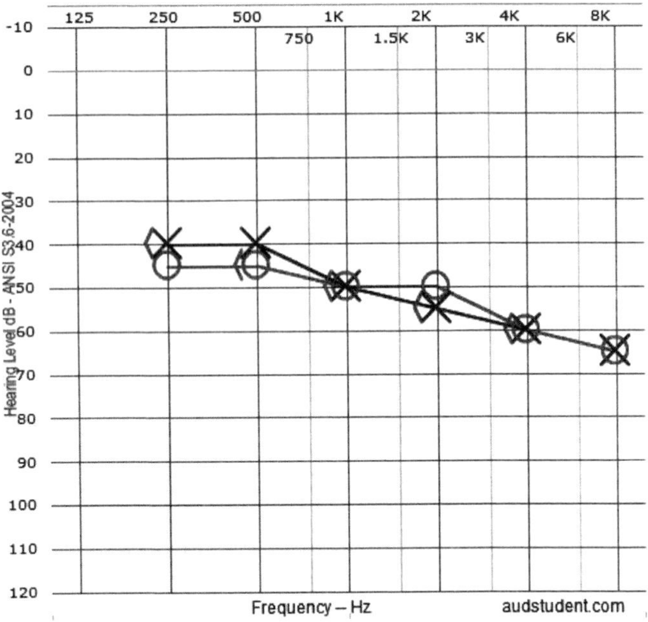

Figure 26–17. Example audiogram for strial involvement from diabetes and cardiovascular disease.

SKULL CONTENT DISORDER: INTRACRANIAL HYPERTENSION

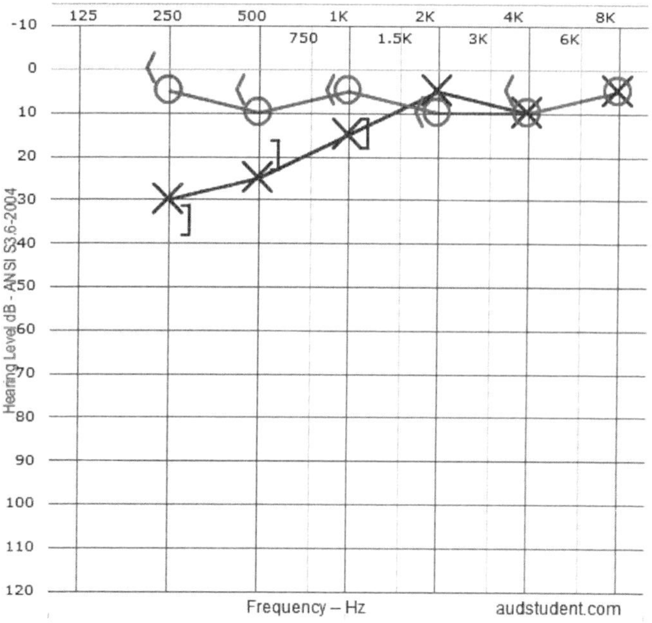

Figure 26–18. Example audiogram for intracranial hypertension.

27

Medical Referral Criteria

OVERVIEW

Steiger (2005) proposed an outline of audiometric referral criteria for audiologists. Below we repeat, update, and expand on those criteria.

CRITERIA FOR MEDICAL CLEARANCE FOR HEARING AID FITTINGS

Here we report criteria often used to determine the need for medical clearance for hearing aid fittings. The criteria need not be limited to hearing aid patients; it can serve as a more general screening of the need for medical evaluation. We recommend that the long-accepted FDA (1977) guidelines as the primary consideration of audiologists. The FDA will no longer enforce those guidelines for adults (FDA press release 2016), and as of this writing the outcome at the state level is uncertain. But regardless of legal or regulatory enforcement, the efficacy and sufficiency of the guidelines has been demonstrated for four decades. We also report the more strict guidelines from the American Academy of Otolaryngology Head and Neck Surgery (AAO-HNS, 1993, 1994) and the AAO-HNS (2015) whenever they differ significantly from the FDA criteria. However, we do not recommend strict adherence to AAO-HNS guideline, as they would result in overreferrals.

Refer When History Indicates:

- Active drainage from the ear within the previous 90 days (FDA, 1977) or within the previous 6 months (AAO-HNS, 1993, 1994) Drainage includes blood (AAO-HNS, 2015)
- Sudden or rapidly progressing hearing loss within the previous 90 days (FDA, 1977) or within the previous 6 months (AAO-HNS,1993,1994)
- Acute or chronic dizziness (FDA, 1977) or recurrent episodes of dizziness (AAO-HNS 2015)
- Otalgia or discomfort in the ear (FDA, 1977)
- Child under 18 years of age (FDA, 1977)
- Complaint of hearing impairment with positive history of tuberculosis, syphilis, HIV, Ménière's disease, auto-immune disorder, otosclerosis, von Recklinghausen's neurofibromatosis, or Paget's disease of the bone (AAO-HNS, 1993, 1994) or positive history of ear infections, noise exposure, familial hearing loss, ototoxic medication use, otosclerosis, or head trauma related to onset (AAO-HNS 2015)

Refer When Otoscopy and Examination Indicates:

- Visible congenital or traumatic deformity of the ear (FDA, 1977). We add our own recommendation to include previously undiagnosed tympanic membrane perforations. This finding requires medical referral with a recommendation of dry-ear precautions. Occluded pressure equalization tubes also require medical referral. Tests such as tympanometry, acoustic reflex evaluation, and wideband acoustic immittance can aid assessment as discussed in Chapters 10, 11, 12, and 15 of this text.
- Visible evidence of significant cerumen accumulation or a foreign body in the ear canal (FDA, 1977). *Note.* Cerumen management is now within the audiology scope of practice for most, if not all, states.
- Visualization of blood, pus, cerumen plug, foreign body, or other material in the ear canal (AAO-HNS, 2015)

Refer When Audiologic Evaluation Indicates:

- Unilateral hearing loss of sudden or recent onset within the previous 90 days (FDA, 1977)
    - AAO-HNS (1993, 1994) clarification of unilateral hearing loss was air-conduction pure-tone PTA (500, 1000, 2000, and 3000 Hz) difference of 15 dB or greater. The AAO-HNS (2015) did not identify

test frequencies. The AAO-HNS (2015) also added unilateral or asymmetrically poor word recognition scores defined as a difference between the ears of greater than 15%.

- Bilateral hearing loss greater than 90 dB (AAO-HNS, 1993, 1994), frequencies not specified.
  - AAO-HNS (2015) guidelines were given as hearing loss greater than 30 dB, frequencies not specified, or bilateral word recognition scores poorer than 80% (AAO-HNS, 2015)
- Audiometric air-bone gap of 15 dB or more at 500 Hz, 1000 Hz, and 2000 Hz (FDA, 1977). The AAO-HNS (2015) added unexplained conductive hearing loss or abnormal tympanogram; see Chapters 10 and 11 of this text for a discussion of tympanograms.

CONSIDERATIONS SPECIFIC TO MAGNETIC RESONANCE IMAGING TO RULE OUT VESTIBULAR SCHWANNOMAS

In addition to the criteria above, Welling, Glasscock, Woods, & Jackson (1990) offered criteria more specific to the recommendation for MRI to diagnose retrocochlear disorder, specifically vestibular schwannomas.

History

- Suspicious information obtained by case history might include (Welling, Glasscock, Woods, & Jackson, 1990):
  - Unexplained unilateral or asymmetric hearing loss
  - Persistent unilateral or asymmetric tinnitus or vertigo/dizziness.
  - Aural fullness
  - Facial paralysis, paresis or weakness

Audiologic Evaluation

- Asymmetric pure-tone air-conduction thresholds options:
  - AAO-HNS criteria: The average difference in air-conduction thresholds between ears of 15 dB or greater at 500 Hz, 1000 Hz, 2000 Hz, and 3000 Hz
  - Obholzer, Rea, and Harcourt (2004) recommendations that have sensitivity (97%) higher than the AAO-HNS criteria and specificity (49%) lower than the AAO-HNS criteria:
    - 15 dB threshold difference between ears at two adjacent frequencies for patients with unilateral hearing loss
    - 20 dB threshold difference between ears at two adjacent frequencies for patients with bilateral hearing loss
- Asymmetric word-recognition scores:
  - One analysis option is the Thornton and Raffin (1978) statistical approach to the identification of significant WRS

asymmetry when measured with NU#6 word lists, see Chapter 7 for details.
  - Another analysis option is the AAO-HNS (2015) criterion of a difference between the ears of greater than 15%.
- Additional tests: Audiologists may add other test to their battery, such as rollover, acoustic reflex thresholds, acoustic reflex decay, and auditory brainstem response (ABR). Test battery sensitivity and specificity can be manipulated (Turner, Frazer, & Sheppard, 1984; Turner, 2013). Generally, the more positive tests an audiologist requires to initiate referrals, the lower the test battery sensitivity (yielding higher miss rates) and the higher the test battery specificity (yielding fewer false alarms).

STRIAL AUDIOGRAMS AND CARDIOVASCULAR DISEASE

Sensorineural hearing loss presenting with flat or gently sloping audiogram configurations could be due to microvascular strial damage; Friedland, Cederberg, and Tarima (2009) reported an association between such hearing loss and cardiovascular compromise. Accordingly, these authors opined that patients presenting with such audiograms be considered for evaluation of cardiovascular disease and risk factors.

CONSIDERATIONS SPECIFIC TO SUDDEN SENSORY/NEURAL HEARING LOSS (SSNHL)

Sudden sensory/neural hearing loss warrants *immediate* referral; therefore the definition (AAO-HNS, 2012) of sudden sensory/neural hearing loss suffices as minimal referral criteria.

- Sudden pure-tone threshold decrease of at least 30 decibels (dB)
  - If previous audiograms are not available, unilateral sudden hearing loss can be defined by comparison to the better ear. For bilateral sudden hearing losses without previous audiograms, some uncertainty is inevitable; see discussion of diagnostic certainty below.
- At least at three consecutive test frequencies
- Over no more than 72 hours.

Levels of Diagnostic Certainty

Clinicians are encouraged to adopt more liberal criteria as case history, test results, and clinical judgment indicates. Accordingly, the AAO-HNS (2012, p. 11) guideline gives levels of diagnostic certainty:

- Very certain: The patient had previous audiometric evaluation.
- Certain: The patient had no prior otologic history and feels his or her premorbid hearing was normal bilaterally.
- Fairly certain: The patient had a long-standing hearing problem and reports

that the current episode of SSNHL is subjectively poorer.
- Uncertain: The clinician feels there was some pre-existing hearing loss, but the hearing loss was never documented.

CONSIDERATIONS SPECIFIC TO TINNITUS

Audiologists should identify patients with neural tinnitus who therefore, are candidates for audiologic treatment. Other tinnitus patients are candidates for medical evaluation (ASHA, 2014; Henry, Zuagg, Myers, & Kendall, 2010; AAO-HNS, 2014). Refer for appropriate medical, emergency, or mental health evaluation with:

- Tinnitus of somatic origin, including pulsatile tinnitus.
- Trauma, facial palsy, or sudden hearing loss.
- Mood disorder, suicidal ideation or obvious mental health problems.
- Symptoms associated with movement of head or neck, such as modulation of tinnitus by head, neck, or eye movement.
- Otalgia, otorrhea, malodor, dizziness, and vertigo.

CONSIDERATIONS SPECIFIC TO DIZZINESS

Audiologists should identify patients with benign paroxysmal positional vertigo (BPPV) who therefore, are candidates for audiologic treatment. Other dizziness patients are candidates for medical evaluation (AAO-HNS, 2008; Smouha & Roussos, 1995). Therefore, medical referral should be considered for:

- Patients with findings atypical to BPPV, including symptoms that are not provoked by head position including negative findings with the Dix-Hallpike.
- Patients with BPPV symptoms showing no improvement after two to three canalith repositioning treatments, possibly indicating misdiagnosis of the canal(s) affected by BPPV, or more misdiagnosis of disorder.

SUMMARY FLOW CHART

Figure 27–1 shows our medical referral flow chart.

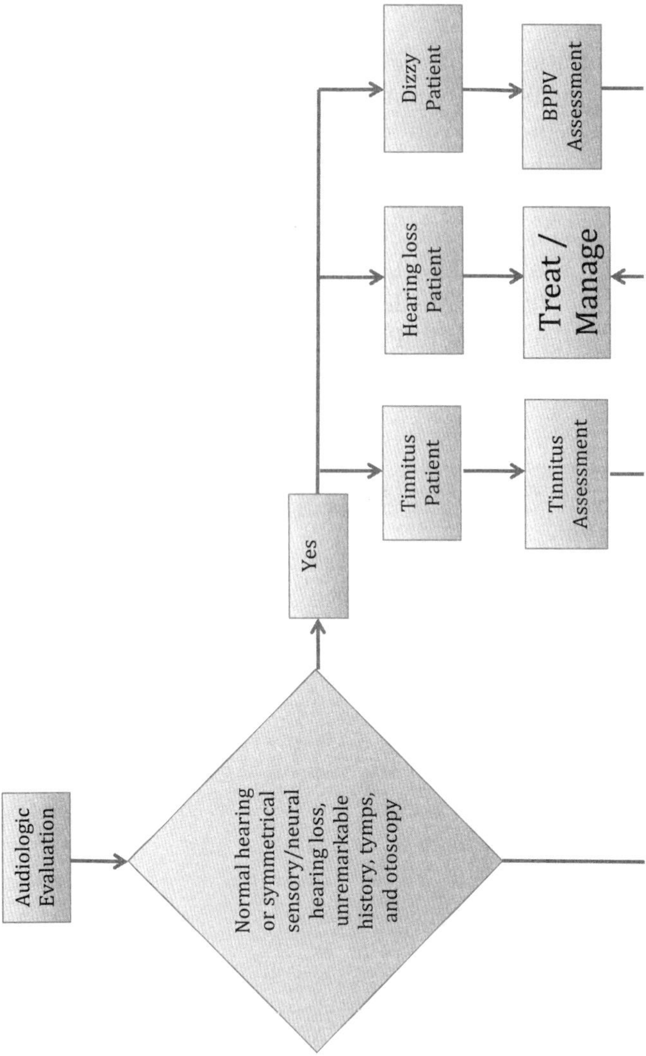
Audiologic Evaluation
Normal hearing or symmetrical sensory/neural hearing loss, unremarkable history, tymps, and otoscopy
Yes
Tinnitus Patient
Hearing loss Patient
Dizzy Patient
Tinnitus Assessment
Treat / Manage
BPPV Assessment

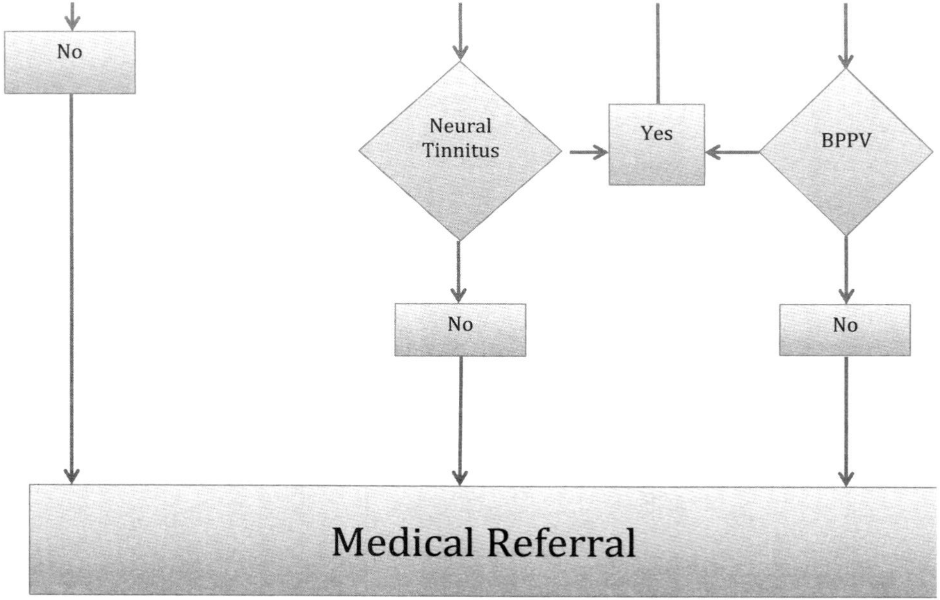

Figure 27–1. Medical referral flow chart.

REFERENCES

American Academy of Otolaryngology-Head and Neck Surgery. (1993). *Bulletin*, 16–17.

American Academy of Otolaryngology-Head and Neck Surgery. (1994). *Bulletin*, 26–28.

American Academy of Otolaryngology-Head and Neck Surgery. (2008). Clinical practice guideline: Benign paroxysmal positional vertigo. *Otolaryngology-Head and Neck Surgery*, *139*(5, Suppl. 4), S47–S81.

American Academy of Otolaryngology-Head and Neck Surgery. (2012). Clinical practice guideline: Sudden hearing loss. *Otolaryngology-Head and Neck Surgery*, *146*, S1–S35. http://dx.doi.org/10.1177/0194599812436449

American Academy of Otolaryngology-Head and Neck Surgery. (2014). Clinical practice guideline: Tinnitus. *Otolaryngology-Head and Neck Surgery*, *151*(Suppl. 2), S1–S40.

American Academy of Otolaryngology-Head and Neck Surgery. (2015). *Position statement: Red flags-warning of ear disease.* Retrieved from http://www.entnet.org/content/position-statement-red-flags-warning-ear-disease

American Speech-Language-Hearing Association. (2014). *Tinnitus triage guidelines: Information for audiologists.* Retrieved from http://www.asha.org/aud/Articles/Tinnitus-Triage-Guidelines/

Food and Drug Administration. (1977). *Hearing aid devices; Professional and patient labeling*. Washington, DC: Government Printing Office.

Friedland, D.R., Cederberg, C., & Tarima, S. (2009). Audiometric pattern as a predictor of cardiovascular status: Development of a model for assessment of risk. *Laryngoscope*, *119*(3), 473–486.

Henry, J. A., Zaugg, T. L., Myers, P. J., & Kendall, C. J. (2010). *Progressive tinnitus management: Clinical handbook for audiologists*. San Diego, CA: Plural.

Obholzer, R. J., Rea, P. A., & Harcourt, J.P. (2004). Magnetic resonance imaging screening for vestibular schwan-

noma: Analysis of published protocols. *Journal of Laryngology and Otology*, *118*(5), 329–332.
Smouha, E. E., & Roussos C. (1995). Atypical forms of paroxysmal positional nystagmus. *Ear Nose and Throat Journal*, *74*(9), 649–656.
Steiger, J. R., (2005). Audiologic referral criteria: Sample clinic guidelines. *Hearing Journal*, *58*(5), 38–42.
Thornton, A. R., & Raffin, M. J. (1978). Speech-discrimination scores modeled as a binomial variable. *Journal of Speech and Hearing Research*, *21*(3), 507–518.
Turner, R. G. (2013). Understanding protocol performance: Impact of criterion and test correlation. *Journal of the American Academy of Audiology*, *24*(10), 897–908.
Turner, R. G., Frazer, G. J., & Sheppard, S. T. (1984). Formulating and evaluation audiologic test protocols. *Ear and Hearing*, *4*(6), 321–330.
U.S. Food and Drug Administration. (2016). *FDA takes steps to improve hearing aid accessibility*. Retrieved from http://www.fda.gov/NewsEvents/Newsroom/PressAnnouncements/ucm532005.htm
Welling, D. B., Glasscock, M. E., Woods, C. L., & Jackson, C. G. (1990). Acoustic neuroma: A cost-effective approach. *Otolarngology-Head and Neck Surgery*, *103*(3), 364–370.

Index

Note: Page numbers in **bold** reference non-text material.

C

D

H

J

K

L

N

P

S

T

W

X

Y

Z

NOTES

NOTES

NOTES

NOTES

NOTES

NOTES

NOTES

NOTES

NOTES

NOTES

NOTES

NOTES

NOTES

NOTES

NOTES

NOTES

NOTES

NOTES

NOTES

NOTES

NOTES

NOTES

NOTES

NOTES